BEYOND HORMONES
7 HOLISTIC WAYS TO THRIVE THROUGH MENOPAUSE

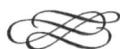

CLARISSA KRISTJANSSON

© Copyright Clarissa Kristjansson - All rights reserved.
The content contained within this book may not be reproduced, duplicated or transmitted without direct written permission from the author or the publisher.

Under no circumstances will any blame or legal responsibility be held against the publisher, or author, for any damages, reparation, or monetary loss due to the information contained within this book. Either directly or indirectly. You are responsible for your own choices, actions, and results.

Legal Notice:

This book is copyright protected. This book is only for personal use. You cannot amend, distribute, sell, use, quote or paraphrase any part, or the content within this book, without the consent of the author or publisher.

Disclaimer Notice:

Please note the information contained within this document is for educational and entertainment purposes only. All effort has been executed to present accurate, up to date, and reliable, complete information. No warranties of any kind are declared or implied. Readers acknowledge that the author is not engaging in the rendering of legal, financial, medical or professional advice. The content within this book has been derived from various sources. Please consult a licensed professional before attempting any techniques outlined in this book.

By reading this document, the reader agrees that under no circumstances is the author responsible for any losses, direct or indirect, which are incurred as a result of the use of the information contained within this document, including, but not limited to, errors, omissions, or inaccuracies.

CONTENTS

Introduction   6

1. Mental & Emotional Well-Being   9
2. Managing Weight Gain   27
3. Diet, Nutrition & Gut Health   45
4. Physical Activity & Exercise   71
5. Sleep Management   87
6. Sexual Health & Intimacy   101
7. Positive Aging Through Menopause   113

Conclusion   129
Bibliography   137

For all those who have helped me to bring this book to fruition.

My wonderful podcast guests, who have generously shared their expertise and passion over the last four years, which has laid the foundations for this book.

I would also like to thank the team behind the scenes who have put so much effort into bringing this book to the market.

My partner for his unwavering support.

INTRODUCTION

In my mid-40s, I was appointed into a new senior role. On the outside, I appeared to have it all. A well-paid role, a lovely child and material comfort. But underneath was a different story. My anxiety, exhaustion and low confidence overwhelmed everything. Broken sleep, unexplained weight gain, rosacea, and escalating blood pressure added to the feeling of being on a downward spiral. I was perimenopausal but didn't know it. Then came the panic attack in the office before my new boss.

After I had wiped away the tears, I knew enough was enough. I didn't quite have all the dots joined, but I knew I couldn't go on this way, crushing me from the inside out. I had to make changes to reclaim my fractured mind, improve my diet, start exercising and improve my mindset.

Let's be real: menopause can suck at times. If you're in perimenopause or menopause, and you're sick of being moody, hot flashy, and sleeping poorly and not feeling like yourself anymore. And have no idea which way to turn.

INTRODUCTION

You may have heard that hot flashes, vaginal dryness, brain fog, acne, weight gain, heavy bleeding, insomnia, anxiety, and depression are "normal at this age,". At this point, you've likely consulted search engines, other women, and your doctor. You may have been offered medication, but you are confused about diet, your mental health, and which exercise is best.

I am here to help you take specific, practical steps to start feeling like yourself again (maybe even better) and regain your groove!

In this book, I unpack the science behind lifestyle, stress, and diet as they pertain to menopause so you can make changes that help you feel more like yourself and even better. How to dial in on what you really want and need so you can have more of it - and enjoy a more fulfilling life now. The best ways you can nurture yourself and optimize your mental, spiritual, and physical wellness.

I'm Clarissa Kristjansson, and I help women master menopause. I am a certified third-age women's health coach, energetic nutritionist, qigong and mindfulness practitioner with 30 years of corporate experience driving behavioral change.

When I first entered the industry almost a decade ago. I saw right away that women were expected to suffer through or be medicated and that there was no integrated approach to managing menopause, let alone thriving at this time. I knew back then that I needed to do something about it.

Alongside my work, I started hosting the Thriving Thru Menopause podcast, which in 2023 was rated the number

INTRODUCTION

one holistic menopause podcast and ranked in the top 8 midlife women's podcasts worldwide. I have interviewed over 200 experts, and this wealth of knowledge has been used to create this ultimate guide to managing menopause holistically.

If you are ready to advocate for what's best for your body and health. Get to the root cause of your menopause issues and how to fix them, feel confident again, and have your energy soaring. Then keep reading!

MENTAL & EMOTIONAL WELL-BEING

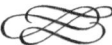

When we talk about menopause, it's easy to focus solely on the physical aspects – the hot flashes, the sleep disturbances, and so on. However, menopause is much more than a series of physical changes; it's a profound journey that encompasses every aspect of our lives. One of the most significant, yet often overlooked, components of this journey is the mental and emotional transition that accompanies it.

This chapter delves into the heart of these mental and emotional shifts. It's common during menopause to experience a roller coaster of emotions, from unexpected bouts of irritability to sudden waves of sadness. These feelings are not just random occurrences; they are deeply intertwined with the hormonal changes taking place in your body. Understanding this connection is the first step towards managing these changes more effectively.

But it's not just about understanding; it's also about acceptance and adaptation. This period of life can be a time of great introspection and personal growth. It offers an opportunity to reassess what truly matters to us and how we want to live our lives moving forward.

As we navigate through these chapters, we'll explore various strategies and practices that can help manage mood swings and emotional turbulence. From mindfulness and meditation to cognitive techniques and building resilience, we'll look at practical ways to foster mental and emotional well-being during menopause.

Menopause is a journey that invites us to rediscover ourselves. It challenges us to find new ways to maintain balance and harmony in our lives. This chapter is here to guide you through that process, offering support and understanding every step of the way.

COPING WITH MOOD SWINGS AND EMOTIONAL CHANGES

Menopause is not just a physical shift; it's a complete neurochemical overhaul. The primary players in this transition are the hormones estrogen and progesterone, whose levels fluctuate significantly during menopause. These hormonal changes are more than just biological markers; they have a profound impact on your emotional state.

Estrogen, in particular, is closely linked to the production and regulation of serotonin, a neurotransmitter often referred to as the 'feel-good hormone'. Serotonin plays a crucial role in mood regulation, and its levels are directly influenced by estrogen. As menopause progresses and estrogen levels decline, so too can serotonin levels, leading to mood swings and emotional fluctuations. Progesterone, known for its calming effects, also decreases during menopause. This decline can result in heightened feelings of anxiety and irritability. Together, the fluctuations of these hormones create a sort of emotional rollercoaster, making you feel like you're losing grip on your once-stable moods.

The brain's limbic system, the emotional center, is highly sensitive to these hormonal changes. As estrogen and progesterone levels fluctuate, so does the activity in the limbic system, leading to varying emotional responses. This sensitivity can make you feel like you're on an emotional pendulum, swinging from joy to sadness with little warning. Additionally, the prefrontal cortex – the part of the brain responsible for decision-making and emotional regulation – also responds to these hormonal changes. This response can affect your ability to manage stress and can lead to feelings of being overwhelmed or unable to cope with everyday challenges.

While hormones play a significant role, it's crucial to acknowledge that external factors also contribute to these mood swings. Life stressors such as career changes, family dynamics, and personal relationships can all intertwine with hormonal fluctuations, exacerbating emotional responses. Understanding this interplay is key to recognizing why you might be feeling more sensitive or irritable than usual.

But it's not all about hormones. Our lives are like intricate tapestries, with threads of career, family, and personal relationships all woven in. These factors can tangle up with our hormonal changes, making our emotional responses even more intense. Recognizing this complex mix can help us understand why we might be feeling extra sensitive or quick to anger.

So, when you're riding this menopausal roller coaster, remember it's not just you – it's a natural part of this transition. Understanding what's going on inside can be the first step to regaining a sense of balance.

RECOGNIZING AND ACKNOWLEDGING EMOTIONS

Let's be honest, menopause can feel like you're on an emotional roller coaster, blindfolded. One moment you're up, the next you're down, and sometimes you're just hanging on for dear life. It's completely normal, and the first step to finding some balance is recognizing and acknowledging these emotions. Think of it as getting to know a new aspect of yourself.

During menopause, your emotions might feel more intense. One minute you're laughing, and the next, you might find tears streaming down your face without any apparent reason. It's okay. These feelings are part of the journey, and recognizing them is like saying, "Hey, I see you, and it's alright to feel this way."

Self-awareness is like your internal compass during menopause. It's about tuning in and really listening to what's going on inside you. When a wave of irritation or a sudden bout of sadness hits, take a moment. Ask yourself gently, "What's really going on here?" Often, these emotions are like icebergs – there's more beneath the surface. Maybe that irritation isn't just about the spilled coffee; perhaps it's the stress of juggling work and life, amplified by the hormonal tango happening in your body.

It's also about recognizing the physical side of these emotions. If you're feeling unusually down, it might be linked to a night of restless sleep or a skipped meal. Menopause can be a bit of a tightrope walk, and acknowledging these physical links can help you find your balance.

Approaching your emotions with curiosity instead of judgment can be a game-changer. In a world that often misunderstands menopause, it's easy to fall into the trap of self-criticism. But beating yourself up over feeling emotional is like getting mad at the weather for raining – it's not something you can control, and it's not your fault. Instead, be kind to yourself. Remind yourself that these emotions are not just 'hormonal episodes'; they're a part of your story.

Have you tried keeping an emotional journal? It's like creating a map of your emotional world. Jotting down how you're feeling and what's happening around you can reveal patterns you might not have noticed. It's empowering, really. You start to see the links, the triggers, and suddenly, you're not just reacting to your emotions; you're understanding them. And with understanding comes a sense of control and peace.

PRACTICAL TIPS FOR IMMEDIATE RELIEF

Navigating menopause is a bit like being an explorer in uncharted territory – exciting but sometimes overwhelming. When those emotional waves hit, it's helpful to have some go-to strategies for immediate relief. These aren't magic cures, but they're like little life rafts that can help you stay afloat during those high-tide moments.

Let's start with something you always have with you – your breath. Deep breathing is like hitting the pause button on life's remote control. It's simple, but oh-so-effective. When you feel a mood swing coming on, take a moment to focus on your breathing. Inhale deeply through your nose, filling your lungs completely, and then exhale slowly through your mouth. Imagine breathing out the stress, the anxiety, the overwhelming emotions. Just a few deep breaths can work wonders in calming your mind and resetting your emotional state.

Next up, short walks. There's something about being outside, feeling the breeze, and taking in the sights and sounds of nature that can be incredibly soothing. It doesn't have to be a long hike – just a brief stroll around your garden or down the street can make a big difference. It's like giving your mind a mini-vacation from the chaos of emotions. Plus, a little bit of physical activity releases those endorphins, nature's feel-good chemicals.

Remember those hobbies you love but never seem to have time for? They're not just fun activities; they're powerful tools for emotional relief. Whether it's painting, gardening, knitting, or playing music, immersing yourself in a hobby can provide a much-needed distraction from mood swings. It's about doing something that brings you joy, something that engages your mind and hands. When you're focused on creating something or doing an activity you love, there's little room for stress and anxiety. It's like stepping into a world where menopause doesn't dictate how you feel.

Lastly, never underestimate the power of connection. Sometimes, when you're riding the menopausal emotional roller coaster, what you really need is to talk to someone who gets it. Reach out to a friend, a family member, or even a support group. Share your feelings, your struggles, and your triumphs. Just talking about what you're going through can be incredibly cathartic. It's a reminder that you're not alone on this journey.

MINDFULNESS PRACTICES: GROUNDING EMOTIONS IN THE MIDST OF CHANGE

Picture menopause like walking through a bustling, lively market – there's so much going on. Mindfulness? It's your quiet corner in that market. It's where you can stop for a moment, take a deep breath, and just be. It's about really being in the moment, feeling life as it happens, not getting tangled up in yesterday or worrying about tomorrow.

During menopause, emotions can swing wildly – one minute you're fine, the next, you're not. Practicing mindfulness is like learning to watch these emotional swings without getting knocked off your feet. It's like watching clouds drift across the sky. They're there, but they don't have to rule your sky. This can mean less stress, a better mood, and it can even take the edge off things like hot flashes.

Simple Mindfulness in Your Day:

Morning Moments: Instead of leaping out of bed each morning, why not take a few minutes just to lie there? Feel the bed beneath you, listen to the sounds around you, breathe deeply. It's like setting the tone for your day – calm and centered.

Eating with Attention: Pick one meal a day and really focus on it. Eat slowly, savor each bite. Notice the textures, the flavors, the colors. It turns a meal into a moment of mindfulness.

Mindful Movement: Whether it's a gentle walk or some stretches, pay attention to how your body feels as you move. Notice the rhythm of your breathing, the way your feet touch the ground, the feeling in your muscles. It's about being present in your movement.

Meditation can be like a calm harbor in the stormy seas of menopause. It's a way to step back from everything and find a bit of peace.

Guided Meditation: There are so many great apps and online resources for this. It's like having someone guide you to a place of calm. They can be great for helping with sleep or just bringing a moment of tranquility into your day.

Sitting with the Moment: This is about sitting quietly, focusing on your breath, and just observing what's happening in your mind and body. Over time, it can help you see what triggers your stress and how to deal with it more calmly.

Remember, the key to both mindfulness and meditation is just to start – even a few minutes each day can make a big difference. Find what works for you and make it a regular part of your life. It's like giving yourself a little gift of peace every day.

COGNITIVE BEHAVIORAL TECHNIQUES: NAVIGATING THE MIND'S PATHWAYS

Imagine your mind as a garden. Over the years, certain paths – your thought patterns – have become well-trodden. Some of these paths are helpful, but others, especially those trodden during menopause, can lead to negative spaces. Cognitive Behavioral Techniques (CBT) are gardening tools, helping you to cultivate healthier pathways in your mental landscape.

The first step is to become aware of these negative thought patterns. For instance, during menopause, you might frequently think, "I'm just getting old and irrelevant." This thought is like a weed in your garden, and acknowledging it is like spotting it amongst your flowers.

Once identified, the next step is to challenge these thoughts. Ask yourself, "Is this really true? Does getting older necessarily mean becoming irrelevant?" This process is like pulling out those weeds and examining them. More often than not, you'll find that these negative thoughts are based on unfounded fears or societal stereotypes.

The final step is to reframe these thoughts into more positive and realistic ones. Instead of thinking, "Menopause is the end of my youthful days," try reframing it to, "Menopause is a new chapter with its own joys and opportunities." This reframing is like planting new seeds in your garden, seeds that will grow into beautiful, positive thoughts.

Examples of Reframing

From: "I can't handle these menopausal changes."

To: "I'm learning to adapt to changes in my body and finding new ways to embrace this phase of life."

From: "Menopause makes me feel less feminine."

To: "Menopause is a natural part of being a woman, and my femininity is defined by more than my reproductive capabilities."

Integrating CBT into Daily Life

CBT isn't an overnight fix. It's a practice, like tending to a garden. It requires time, patience, and regular maintenance. You can practice these techniques on your own, or, for more guided assistance, consider working with a therapist specializing in CBT. Over time, you'll notice your mental garden flourishing with positive, empowering thoughts.

AROMATHERAPY: EMPOWERMENT THROUGH SMELL

Aromatherapy is a holistic healing treatment that uses natural plant extracts to promote health and well-being. Using essential oils during menopause can be incredibly beneficial - they can have a profound impact on our limbic system, the part of the brain that controls emotions, behaviors, and even long-term memory. This is why a certain scent can suddenly bring back a flood of memories or impact our mood so strongly. They are like the fragrant allies in our menopause toolkit, helping us manage stress and improve our mood.

Let's dive into some specific essential oils and how they can help us during menopause:

- Lavender: Ah, the classic! Lavender is like a gentle hug for your nervous system. It's renowned for its relaxation properties. Having trouble sleeping? Feeling a bit anxious? Lavender oil can be your go-to. Use it in a diffuser in your bedroom, or add a few drops to a warm bath before bedtime. It's like enveloping yourself in a calming, soothing blanket.Peppermint: Need a pick-me-up? Peppermint oil is your friend. It's energizing and refreshing – perfect for those sluggish mornings or afternoon slumps. You can dab a little on your wrists or temples (be careful to dilute it with a carrier oil if you have sensitive skin), or simply inhale it for a quick energy boost.
- Clary Sage: This oil is particularly good for balancing hormones, making it a fantastic choice for menopausal women. Clary sage can help alleviate hot flashes and promote emotional balance. Mix it with a carrier oil and massage it into your skin, or use it in a diffuser to create a balancing atmosphere in your home or office.

- Geranium: Known for its ability to enhance mood and balance hormones, geranium oil is like a multi-tool in your menopause kit. It's great for everything from mood swings to dry skin. Use it in your skincare routine, or diffuse it to create a pleasant, uplifting environment.
- Ylang Ylang: This exotic oil is a powerful mood lifter. It can help combat depression and anxiety, which are common during menopause. Plus, it's known for its libido-boosting properties. Ylang Ylang's sweet, floral scent makes it a delightful addition to your self-care routine.

You can use these oils in various ways: diffuse them, apply them topically (always diluted with a carrier oil), or simply inhale them directly from the bottle. They can be blended for a more complex scent and therapeutic effect, or used individually for a more targeted approach. Think of aromatherapy not just as an immediate relief tactic, but as a form of self-expression during menopause. In the interest of making your menopausal journey as pleasant and empowering as possible, why not explore the world of essential oils and discover the scents that speak to your soul during this transformative time?

BUILDING RESILIENCE: EMBRACING THE WAVES OF CHANGE

Think of resilience as the ability to be flexible and adapt to change, like a tree that bends in the wind but doesn't break. Menopause, with all its challenges, offers a unique opportunity to strengthen this ability. It's about embracing change – not just enduring it, but finding strength and growth in the experience.

Change, especially during menopause, can often feel daunting. Hot flashes, mood swings, and all the other fun stuff can sometimes make you feel like you're losing your footing. But here's the thing: these changes are not just obstacles; they're stepping stones to a more resilient you.

One way to build resilience is to shift your perspective. Instead of viewing menopause as a series of losses (loss of youth, loss of fertility), try seeing it as a series of gains – wisdom, experience, and perhaps a newfound sense of freedom. This shift in perspective can transform the way you experience menopause, turning it from a time of dread to a period of discovery.

Your menopause journey is uniquely yours, but it's also a shared experience with millions of other women. There's strength in that. Recognize that each hot flash, each sleepless night, is a shared rite of passage. It's a natural part of life, not a flaw or a failure.

Building resilience also means being kind to yourself. Be as compassionate to yourself as you would be to a friend going through the same changes. Allow yourself the time to adapt, the space to grow, and the grace to not always get it right.

Remember to celebrate the small victories. Made it through a meeting without a hot flash? That's a win. Managed to laugh instead of snapping during an emotional wave? Another win. These small triumphs are markers of your resilience, signs that you're adapting and growing.

POSITIVE COPING STRATEGIES: NURTURING YOUR WELL-BEING

Navigating menopause can feel like you're charting a course through uncharted waters. It's full of surprises and changes, and having some positive coping strategies is like having a reliable compass to guide you through. These aren't just strategies to get you through the tough moments; they're about bringing joy, creativity, and a sense of connection into your everyday life.

Journaling: Your Heart on Paper

Journaling during menopause is more than just writing down words; it's like having a heartfelt chat with a dear friend. Imagine pouring out all those swirling thoughts and emotions onto paper. This process can be incredibly cathartic. It's a safe space where you can express your fears, celebrate your triumphs, and reflect on your journey without any filters or judgments. Plus, when you start noticing patterns in what you write, it can be a real eye-opener. You might discover what triggers those mood swings or what brings a sense of calm, giving you valuable insights into managing your menopausal journey better.

Connecting Through Support Groups

Think of support groups as your personal cheer squad. They're spaces filled with other women who are riding the same rollercoaster as you. Sharing your stories, tips, or even a few good laughs can be incredibly uplifting. These groups remind you that you're not navigating this journey alone. There's something quite powerful about being in a room (virtual or otherwise) with people who really get what you're going through. It's a mix of empathy, shared wisdom, and genuine understanding that can make all the difference on tough days.

Crafting a Wellness Plan That Lasts

Looking beyond the immediate challenges of menopause, it's important to plan for your long-term wellness. This is about creating a blueprint for a life filled with health, happiness, and fulfillment.

Staying Active in Ways You Love

Integrating regular physical activity into your life is crucial, but it's not about forcing yourself through workouts that you dread. It's about discovering activities that you genuinely enjoy. Perhaps it's a dance class that fills you with energy, a yoga session that brings you peace, or nature walks that connect you with the outdoors. The key is to find joy in movement, making it something you look forward to rather than a chore. Regular physical activity not only helps in managing menopausal symptoms but also boosts your overall health – strengthening bones, improving cardiovascular health, and enhancing mental well-being.

Keeping Connected

Maintaining social connections is as vital as a balanced diet for your emotional health. Regular interactions with friends, family, and community can provide a support network, reduce feelings of isolation, and increase your sense of belonging. Whether it's regular catch-ups with friends, joining a book club, or volunteering for a cause you're passionate about, these connections can bring laughter, joy, and a sense of community into your life.

Embracing Learning and New Hobbies

Finally, keep your curiosity alive. Menopause can be the perfect time to explore new hobbies or revisit old ones. Maybe there's a language you've always wanted to learn, a craft you've wanted to try, or a subject you're curious about. Embracing lifelong learning and new hobbies isn't just about keeping busy; it's about enriching your life, stimulating your mind, and finding joy in discovery. This pursuit of learning and hobbies can bring a new sense of purpose and fulfillment to your life.

CONCLUSION

Wrapping up this chapter, we've really dived deep into the emotional waves that come with menopause. It's clear that this journey isn't just about hot flashes or night sweats; it's also about the whirlwind of feelings stirring inside us. We've shed light on the hormonal ballet affecting our moods and looked into a toolbox full of strategies to keep our emotional ship steady. From mindfulness to belly laughs with friends, and from the grounding power of aromatherapy to the clarity brought by cognitive techniques, we've explored ways to not just survive but thrive through these changes. It's all about turning menopause from something we just have to deal with, into a chance to really get to know ourselves better and make the most out of every day!

Chapter Takeaways:

- The hormonal fluctuations of menopause significantly impact our emotional well-being, highlighting the importance of understanding this neurochemical overhaul.
- Acknowledging and addressing the emotional rollercoaster of menopause is key to fostering mental resilience and stability.
- Practical strategies, including mindfulness, aromatherapy, and cognitive behavioral techniques, offer immediate relief and long-term benefits for managing mood swings and emotional turbulence.
- Cultivating a supportive community, and adopting a holistic approach to wellness can profoundly influence our fulfilment through menopause.

Recommended listening for this chapter from the Thriving Thru Menopause Podcast:

- Season 2 Episode 8: Empowering Women in Menopause
- Season 2 Episode 16: Are You Ready to Say Goodbye to Anxiety
- Season 5 Episode 23: Self-Compassion & Menopause

Scan This QR Code To Listen On Your Favorite Podcast App

MANAGING WEIGHT GAIN

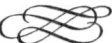

You're eating and exercising the same as always but your body decides to change the rules just when you thought you had it all figured out. The decrease in estrogen and progesterone in perimenopause, along with aging in general, triggers changes in the body.

We used to think that was due to a slowing metabolism but a 2021 study published in *Science* found that this change in weight isn't due to slowing metabolism like we once thought - and that other factors are contributing to weight gain.

One change is a decrease in muscle mass, resulting in fewer calories being burned. If fewer calories are being burned, fat accumulates. Genetics and environmental factors like a lack of sleep, a calorically dense diet, heightened stress response and a sedentary lifestyle, are important considerations. It can be a vicious cycle. We lose muscle tone and accumulate more fat as we age, contributing to more weight gain. And that cycle continues.

This isn't just about a few extra pounds; it's about how our body composition shifts. We might notice more fat around the belly. It's like our bodies are holding onto those calories for dear life.

HORMONAL IMBALANCE AND FAT DISTRIBUTION

Now, let's talk about where this weight tends to show up. During menopause, fat has a way of redistributing itself – and not where we want it. We're talking more around the abdomen, less on the hips and thighs. This isn't just a matter of fitting into your jeans; it's about health. The type of fat that makes up our menopause belly is called Visceral Fat and it covers our organs and increases the risk of diabetes, heart disease, high blood pressure, stroke and respiratory problems. Also, the extra weight on the joints leads to arthritic issues that limit mobility and make it harder to exercise

In perimenopause, a decrease in the production of estrogen and progesterone occurs, which plays a major role in blood sugar fluctuations. Insulin is a hormone produced by the pancreas that helps the body use glucose for the fuel it needs and stores the rest. Estrogen optimizes insulin activity in the body. The decline of estrogen levels makes way for insulin resistance and spikes in blood sugar levels, leading to crashes and cravings.

While progesterone impacts our sleep and ability to manage stress and its rapid decline in perimenopause spawns a cluster of symptoms that directly impact blood sugar levels.

The honest truth is you can't tolerate sugar as well as you did when you were younger. Low estrogen levels reduce sensitivity to insulin which means that you cannot clear sugar from the blood as efficiently and this increases your risk of type 2 diabetes, weight gain and poor mood.

NUTRITIONAL STRATEGIES FOR WEIGHT MANAGEMENT: FINDING YOUR BALANCE

Managing weight during menopause isn't just about what the scale says; it's about creating harmony in your body through what you eat. It is time to forget all the dieting - put simply diets don't work! And that can be hard if you're like most women; you've probably spent decades on diets. Heck, some women have done 60 different diets by the time perimenopause hits.

We have programmed so that our natural response to this weight gain is often to start restricting what we eat. A huge number of women simply aren't eating enough. 900 calories, way too many women attempt to survive on, is barely sufficient for your body to meet its basic needs. And it makes the belly fat worse. The poor body is tipped into starvation mode, and it holds onto every calorie for dear life.

What works best for maintaining a healthy weight is a balanced diet with sufficient calories. Choose foods that take longer to digest. Studies show that a low-glycemic index diet may be beneficial for managing weight and blood sugar levels associated with menopause.

Picture your meals as a vibrant mix of colors and textures, with plenty of vegetables, good proteins, and healthy fats.

This isn't a calorie-counting game; it's about giving your body the nutrients it needs to stay within a healthy weight.

Fiber-rich foods, like your leafy greens, whole grains, and beans, are fantastic for keeping you full and satisfied. They're the kind of foods that do double duty – they keep your hunger at bay and support your overall health. These foods are high in soluble fiber and slow gastric emptying. That means it keeps you fuller for longer. One study found that for every 10-gram increase in soluble fiber daily, belly fat was reduced by 3.7%. Soluble fiber is found in cruciferous vegetables, beans, avocados, oats, nuts and seeds. Ten grams of soluble fiber equates to having half an avocado on whole-grain toast for breakfast, adding beans to lunch, and pairing a protein at dinner with a side of Brussels sprouts.

Spotlight on Key Nutrients

In the world of nutrients, some are particularly beneficial during menopause. And the most important as we age is protein. Higher protein intake is linked to increased lean body mass in postmenopausal women. Studies addressing belly fat found that a low carbohydrate, higher protein dietary combination may yield the most effective results. Consuming protein throughout the day will help ensure you're hitting the daily recommendation. For example, consider yogurt with nuts and berries for breakfast, a bean-based soup for lunch, cheese and an apple for a snack, and wild salmon and greens for dinner.

Increase your phytoestrogens to help with the hormonal roller coaster. Phytoestrogens are found in plants, and they help top up our estrogens in a very weak form and can help support insulin sensitivity and other metabolic changes. You can find them in soya-based foods such as tofu, tempeh, and edamame beans as well as ground flaxseed broccoli, cabbage, and cauliflower.

Consider adding shelled edamame as a snack, tempeh as a protein source on salads or miso soup as an appetizer to a meal.

Portion Sizes and Meal Timing

As for portion sizes and when you eat, it's about finding a rhythm that works for you. You don't need to eat tiny amounts, but it's about eating enough to fuel your body without overdoing it. Regular, well-balanced meals can help keep your energy levels steady throughout the day and keep those intense cravings at bay.

When it comes to portion sizes, think of it as finding the perfect fit for your body. It's not about piling your plate high or measuring out every morsel, but rather tuning into your body's hunger cues. A good rule of thumb is to start with smaller servings. You can always go back for seconds if you're still hungry, but often you'll find that your eyes are bigger than your stomach. Visual cues can be really helpful here. For instance, a serving of protein should be about the size of your palm, and a serving of carbs, like rice or pasta, should be about the size of your clenched fist. Fill the rest of your plate with vegetables, aiming for variety and color. This approach helps with portion control and ensures you're getting a good balance of nutrients.

Lose the booze. One habit that significantly improves weight management is limiting alcohol intake. The data on alcohol is clear, it can disrupt sleep and add excess calories. Having more than three drinks on any day seven to eight drinks per week, poses a risk to both health and weight. Limiting alcohol to a few days per week may assist with weight management.

Timing Your Meals for Metabolic Health

As for meal timing, it's about creating a rhythm that supports your metabolism and keeps your energy levels steady throughout the day. Skipping meals can lead you to become ravenous and overeat later, so try to eat at regular intervals.

A good practice is to have a hearty breakfast – it kick starts your metabolism and gives you the energy you need to start the day. Then, listen to your body for cues on lunch and dinner. Try not to eat too late in the evening, as your body's metabolism slows down at night, making it harder to digest food.

Remember, it's also about being responsive to your body. Some days, you might need a bit more; other days, a bit less, and that's okay. It's about finding what works for you and being flexible. And don't forget to drink water throughout the day. Sometimes we mistake thirst for hunger, so staying well-hydrated can also help manage your appetite.

NAVIGATING THE CRAVING MAZE DURING MENOPAUSE

Let's face it, one of the biggest surprises that menopause brings along is the bunch of cravings you didn't expect. One minute you're fine, and the next, you're daydreaming about chocolate, a bag of chips, or a big, fluffy piece of bread. Common menopause symptoms can have us reaching for those sugary snacks. But, have you ever stopped to think that maybe these cravings aren't just about hunger? Sometimes, they're more like emotional signals in disguise. Fatigue, mood swings, hot flashes and lack of sleep have us reaching for a quick fix as the body searches for quick energy. This is why when you are running on empty and feel depleted, sugar cravings might start to feel unmanageable. Simple carbs provide a short-term boost but are soon followed by a 'crash' leading to more cravings and starting the cycle again!

If you find yourself reaching for a snack, opt for something that combines a bit of protein, healthy fats, and fiber. This could be a small handful of nuts and a piece of fruit, or some carrot sticks with hummus. These kinds of snacks are satisfying and can help tide you over until your next meal.

Beyond satisfying your snacking needs with food, understanding why you get your sugar cravings is the first step to quitting. If you know you are comforting yourself, consider what else might help that isn't food-related. If it's down to boredom, what could you do instead to fill your time?

It's like your body is using food cravings to wave a flag, saying "Hey, something's up!" But often, it's not really the food it's after. Maybe it's boredom, stress, or some pent-up emotions looking for an outlet. It is also important to recognise that lack of sleep increases these cravings. When we are over tired our brain ignores the appetite suppressor, leptin, we develop a resistance that allows our appetite stimulator hormone ghrelin to run riot.

That's where a food diary can be so, so helpful along with getting our sleep on track (more on this in Chapter 5). We're trying to use the food diary in a similar way a detective uses their notebook. Each entry helps you unravel the mystery of your cravings. When you jot down what you eat, also note what you're feeling or what's happening around you. Were you feeling lonely, anxious, or maybe just tired? Over time, this diary will reveal patterns – like maybe you reach for sweets more often when you're stressed, or salty snacks become irresistible when you're bored.

With these insights, you can start finding ways to address the real issue. If it's stress, maybe a quick walk or some deep breaths could help. If it's boredom, how about calling a friend or diving into a good book? It's about finding healthier responses to these emotional cues.

Remember, managing cravings during menopause is as much about understanding your emotions as it is about controlling what you eat. It's a journey of self-discovery, where you learn to listen to and care for both your body and your emotional well-being.

INCORPORATING REGULAR PHYSICAL ACTIVITY AND STRENGTH TRAINING

90% of weight management is diet but exercise is critical. And the calories in calories out model will not work so starving yourself and doing loads of cardio will not shift that meno-belly. But exercise of the right kind is like giving your metabolism a helpful nudge, keeping it active and efficient. Regular exercise doesn't just help with weight management; it also boosts your mood and energy levels. Think of it as your natural energy drink, minus the sugar crash.

Now, strength training deserves a special mention. Too many women often stick to cardio, sometimes because we feel less comfortable in the weights section of the gym. Time to forget the Jane Fonda leggings and all and embrace those weights.

As we age, our muscle mass naturally starts to decline, this is known as sarcopenia, which can slow down our metabolism. It's like the engine of your car running on low gear. Strength training is your tool to rev up that engine. By maintaining and building muscle mass, you also ensure that your metabolism stays fired up. Think of it like putting money in a high savings account that works in the gym or when you're chilling by the pool.

Incorporating exercises like weight lifting, resistance band workouts, or body-weight exercises like squats and push-ups can make a significant difference. It's not about becoming a bodybuilder; it's about giving your body the strength it needs to function at its best.

Creating an exercise routine that you can stick to is like building a bridge to your future self – the one who's healthier, fitter, and happier. Most guidelines recommend aiming for 150 minutes of exercise per week. But for many of us this isn't where we are. The good news is that women who did 10 minutes of exercise a day can remove six inches smaller around the waist than those who didn't exercise. That should be an inspiration to get moving.

A great fitness and movement formula for women as we age that positively impacts bone health, builds muscle and improves CV health means mixing strength and stamina-type exercises that can include cardiovascular exercises (like walking, swimming, or cycling) that increase your heart rate, along with strength training with weights and resistance bands. Plus add in flexibility workouts (like yoga or Pilates) because we tend to stiffen up as we get into menopause thanks to a drop in estrogen, which also plays a role in keeping us supple.

Start small. Walking is a great place to start, 20 minutes a day of walking at a slower pace until you find your stride but try your best to ramp up your pace every week or so to help continue to make progress toward your weight loss goals. And, if you're looking for a more challenging walking workout, try incorporating hills or an incline (if you're working out on a treadmill) to burn some additional calories.

If you are just starting out then using your own body weight to strength train and tame belly fat during menopause is great. Forearm planks, and push ups on your knees are all good.

Then you can incorporate free weights. If you're just starting out, lighter, 2–5-pound, free weights are probably best and these can even be tins from your cupboards or bottle of water. Work up to the gym or find an online training programme, maybe run by someone who specializes in helping menopausal women.

The key is consistency and finding a balance that keeps you motivated. It's also okay to start small and gradually increase the intensity and duration of your workouts. Remember, this is a marathon, not a sprint.

And lastly, listen to your body. Some days you might need to push a little harder; others, a walk might be enough. It's about finding that sweet spot where exercise feels challenging yet enjoyable.

INTEGRATIVE APPROACHES AND LIFESTYLE MODIFICATIONS

When it comes to managing weight, especially during menopause, stress is like an invisible force that can throw everything off balance. It's not just about the stress of a busy day; it's how this constant pressure can lead to weight gain. Stress triggers the release of cortisol, a hormone that, in excess, can make your body hold onto fat, especially around the belly.

Stress can be a bit of a chameleon, showing up in various ways that we might not immediately link to being stressed out. For many of us in this stage of life, stress can manifest in several common symptoms:

- Sleep Disturbances: You might find yourself tossing and turning at night or waking up at odd hours. This restlessness isn't just about feeling tired; it's a classic sign of stress affecting your sleep cycle.
- Mood Swings: Sure, mood swings can be a part of menopause, but they're also a big red flag for stress. If you find yourself snapping at minor things or

feeling unexpectedly emotional, stress might be the culprit.
- Physical Symptoms: Stress can show up physically, too. This can range from headaches and muscle tension to digestive issues. It's like your body's alarm system signaling that something's off.
- Fatigue and Low Energy: Feeling like you're constantly running on empty, despite getting enough rest, can be a sign of chronic stress. It's that feeling of being drained, even when you haven't exerted yourself.
- Changes in Appetite or Eating Habits: Stress can mess with your appetite. Some of us might start skipping meals without realizing it, while others might turn to comfort eating.
- Difficulty Concentrating: If you're finding it hard to focus or keep forgetting things, stress might be affecting your cognitive functions.

So, how do we tackle this sneaky stress? First, recognize its presence. Just acknowledging that you're stressed can be a big step. Then, introduce relaxation techniques into your daily routine. This could be as simple as deep breathing exercises, practicing mindfulness, or finding time for activities that bring you joy. And let's not forget to sleep – it's like hitting the reset button for your body and mind. Aim for 7-8 hours of quality sleep each night. It might mean establishing a soothing bedtime routine or making your bedroom a tech-free zone.

When it comes to these lifestyle changes, think of it as a journey, not a sprint. Quick fixes might sound appealing, but they rarely lead to long-term success. It's about making small, sustainable changes that add up over time. For instance, start by swapping out processed foods for whole foods, or by gradually increasing your daily activity level. These changes don't have to be drastic; even small shifts can lead to significant results over time.

MINDFUL EATING

Mindful eating is not just a way of eating; it's a way of living. It's like turning each meal into a mini-meditation, where you're fully in the moment with your food. This practice can transform your relationship with food, turning it from a mindless act into a source of joy and nourishment.

Start by engaging all your senses. Look at your food – notice the colors and shapes on your plate. Take a moment to appreciate the journey this food has taken to reach you. As you take your first bite, tune into the textures and flavors. Is it crunchy or smooth? Sweet, salty, or tangy? Notice the temperature and the sensations in your mouth. Our lives are often a hectic rush, and eating can become just another task to hurry through. Mindful eating invites you to slow down. Chew each bite thoroughly. This not only helps with digestion but also gives you the time to truly taste your food. It's surprising how much more flavorful a meal can be when you eat it slowly.

One of the most significant aspects of mindful eating is learning to recognize your body's signals. Before you start eating, ask yourself how hungry you are on a scale from 1 to 10. Do the same after you've finished eating. This practice helps you tune into your body's true needs, helping you differentiate between true hunger and eating out of boredom or emotion. Mindful eating also means being aware of the emotional aspects of food. Food can be comforting, and that's okay. The key is to recognize when you're eating to fill an emotional void rather than physical hunger. By being mindful, you can start to break the cycle of emotional eating. Start small. Perhaps begin with one mindful meal a day. Turn off the TV, put away your phone, and eliminate distractions. Make this a time for you and your food. As you get more comfortable with this practice, you can start incorporating it into more meals. Mindful eating is a journey, not a destination. It's about continually coming back to the present moment and experiencing your food with all your senses. Over time, this practice can lead to healthier eating habits, improved digestion, and a more joyful relationship with food.

MONITORING PROGRESS AND ADJUSTING GOALS

Keeping track of your progress shows you how far you've come and helps guide where you need to go next. This could be as simple as keeping a food diary, tracking your exercise routine, or regularly checking in on how you feel both physically and emotionally.

Setting realistic goals is also key. Instead of aiming for a drastic weight loss in a short period, set smaller, achievable targets. And be prepared to adjust these goals as needed. Your body and needs can change, especially during menopause, and your goals should reflect this. Remember, this journey is uniquely yours, and what works for someone else might not work for you. It's about finding your path and walking it at your own pace.

CONCLUSION

Navigating weight management during menopause isn't just about counting calories or increasing exercise; it's about understanding the deeper hormonal shifts and how they influence our bodies. In this chapter we've explored the multifaceted relationship between menopause, weight gain, and overall well-being, emphasizing that effective weight management is grounded in a balanced diet, mindful of hormonal health, and complemented by physical activity tailored to your needs. By integrating stress management and adopting lifestyle changes that resonate with our changing bodies, we can approach weight management not as a battle but as an opportunity for nurturing and self-care. Remember, the journey through menopause is uniquely yours, and embracing it with knowledge, patience, and compassion can lead to a fulfilling path of health and vitality.

Chapter Takeaways:

- Acknowledge the impact of decreased estrogen and progesterone on weight gain and fat distribution, focusing on the importance of managing these changes through diet and lifestyle adjustments.
- Embrace a balanced diet rich in fiber, protein, and key nutrients, steering clear of restrictive diets and focusing on nourishing your body.
- Incorporate regular exercise, especially strength training, to maintain muscle mass and metabolism. Start small and build a routine that fits your lifestyle and preferences.
- Recognize stress as a significant factor in weight management, adopting practices like mindfulness, adequate sleep, and relaxation techniques to mitigate its effects.
- Use food diaries and awareness of emotional triggers to navigate cravings effectively, opting for balanced snacks that satisfy nutritional needs.
- Monitor progress and set achievable targets, understanding that flexibility and patience are key to adapting goals as you navigate through menopause.
- Practice mindful eating, engaging with your food on a sensory level, savoring each bite and listening to your body's signals.

Recommended listening for this chapter, from the Thriving Thru Menopause Podcast:

- Season 5 Episode 7: How to Release Weight and Get Your Energy Soaring
- Season 4 Episode 7: The Real Weight- Loss Formula in Midlife? MINDSET

Scan This QR Code To Listen On Your Favorite Podcast App

DIET, NUTRITION & GUT HEALTH

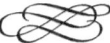

As you journey through menopause, understanding the role of nutrition becomes paramount. This chapter is dedicated to unraveling the complexities of how food can support hormonal balance, mitigate inflammation, and cater to your body's evolving needs. We delve into the power of phytoestrogens, the necessity of optimizing nutrient intake, and making practical dietary adjustments to harmonize with your changing body. Not to mention gut health, something often overlooked yet critical for overall well being in menopause. We'll also unravel just exactly how the gut-brain connection works and how we can keep a healthy gut to promote overall health in menopause.

NUTRITIONAL NEEDS DURING MENOPAUSE FOR HORMONAL BALANCE

Menopause can feel like a bit of a balancing act, especially when it comes to your hormones. But what if your diet could lend a helping hand? But here's where phytoestrogens, naturally occurring compounds in certain foods like soy and flaxseeds, come into play. Phytoestrogens are fascinating because they're similar in structure to the estrogen produced by our bodies. Imagine a lock and key system where estrogen is the key, and estrogen receptors in our body are the locks. Phytoestrogens can fit into these same locks, but they don't turn the lock as strongly as our body's own estrogen. This is why they're often called 'weak estrogens.'

When your body's natural estrogen levels begin to wane during menopause, phytoestrogens can step in and gently activate these estrogen receptors. They don't replace your body's estrogen completely, but they can help fill the gap, reducing the intensity of menopause symptoms. This mimicry of estrogen can be particularly helpful for managing common menopausal symptoms like hot flashes and mood swings. For instance, when phytoestrogens bind to estrogen receptors in the brain, they can help modulate body temperature, which might provide some relief from those sudden, intense waves of heat.

Similarly, by interacting with estrogen receptors in the brain that regulate mood, phytoestrogens can help bring a sense of emotional balance, easing those mood swings that often accompany menopause.

Including phytoestrogen-rich foods in your diet is like having a toolkit for hormone management. Top of the list are soy-based foods. Fermented and whole soybeans contain the highest concentrations of phytoestrogens, and those appear to be the healthiest ways to consume soy. Fermented soy products include miso and tempeh (the latter boasts whole soybeans), edamame and tofu.

Try to buy organic if you can as many of the non-organic soy products are from GMO seeds and heavily sprayed with glyphosate based weed killers. No one wants to be eating bug spray!. Check if you buy soy milk that it doesn't contain a whole load of sugar and seed oils because these inflammatory ingredients counteract any goodness from the beans.

Nuts and seeds are also foods rich in phytoestrogens. Flaxseeds are actually higher in phytoestrogens than soybeans. Also scoring high are pistachios, chestnuts, walnuts, hazelnuts, and cashew. These make great snacks if you are feeling low in energy.

Garlic and onion are no phytoestrogen slouches either when it comes to phytoestrogens. Think winter squash, as well as the cruciferous family, including broccoli, cabbage, and many leafy greens like spinach and kale. You can also find phytoestrogens in fresh fruit, including blueberries, peaches, strawberries, raspberries, and dried fruit such as dates and apricots.

It's important to note that the effects of phytoestrogens can vary depending on individual body chemistry, so they may work differently for different people. As with any dietary change, it's about listening to your body and seeing what works best for you.

OPTIMIZING NUTRIENT INTAKE

Another key piece of the puzzle is ensuring your diet contains sufficient essential vitamins and minerals, so called micronutrients. During menopause, your needs for certain nutrients go up a notch.

Calcium is crucial for maintaining bone health, especially as the risk of osteoporosis increases as we go through menopause. But Vitamin D is the vital piece and without vitamin D, only about 15% of dietary calcium and 60% of phosphorus are absorbed. On the other hand, with enough vitamin D calcium absorption increases by up to 40% and phosphorus absorption increases by 80%.

Vitamin D does a whole lot more. It supports brain health, muscle size and strength, heart health, mood, pancreas health and insulin balance. Although you can get Vitamin D from fifteen to twenty minutes of sunshine daily with more than 40% of your skin exposed. Most people aren't getting enough direct sun exposure - even in the summer - to produce enough vitamin D. To further fracture proof your bones it is recommended to take Vitamin K2 along with your Vitamin D as this will help reverse bone loss, support the growth of stronger bones and reduces fractures more than 80%.

Magnesium plays a vital role in health and in menopause, it's important for keeping bones strong and preventing osteoporosis. Magnesium may also reduce unwanted side effects of menopause, such as difficulty sleeping and depression while supporting heart health. Magnesium is a gentle muscle relaxer and you might experience the benefits by taking some magnesium at bedtime.

Most menopausal women have inadequate magnesium levels, putting them at greater risk of poor health. However, magnesium can be consumed through many foods, such as dark chocolate, beans, lentils, nuts, seeds, leafy greens, and whole grains. But additional supplementation may also be helpful. The forms of magnesium that is most absorbable are the magnesium glycinate, magnesium malate or magnesium amino acid chelate.

And let's not forget the B vitamins – they're vital for energy production, brain health, and managing stress, in particular B6 and B12. B12 is key for protecting your heart and brain, supporting good gut health, and helping your nervous system and eyes work properly. While B6 may help ward off menopausal depression and increase energy by boosting serotonin.

So, how do you pack all these nutrients into your diet? It's about variety and balance. Eating the rainbow is very good advice and if you can try to get 30 different types of plant based foods into your week. It might sound like a lot but remember fruit, veggies, beans, lentils, oats and even herbs and spices all count towards the total.

Enjoy a mix of dairy or fortified non-dairy sources for calcium, get some sunshine for vitamin D, add nuts and leafy greens for magnesium, and don't skimp on those whole grains for the B vitamins. Plus supplementation with high quality supplements can be highly supportive. It's important to remember the cheaper grocery brands are sometimes more filler than micro-nutrients so check the labels and seek out recommendations from a functional doctor or nutritionist if required.

MEDICINAL HERBS

As we've explored the essentials of a balanced diet, rich in phytoestrogens, fibers, and vitamins, let's delve deeper into another key layer of nutrition in menopause: medicinal herbs. In this context, they serve as a botanical compass, offering guidance and relief through nature's own pharmacy. These natural allies provide a gentle yet effective approach to managing menopausal symptoms, aligning with the body's intrinsic processes.

Now, you might be wondering, why herbs? The appeal of medicinal herbs lies in their long-standing history and the wisdom of traditional medicine. Cultures from all corners of the globe have relied on the healing powers of nature long before modern medicine came into play. When it comes to tackling our menopausal symptoms, certain herbs have gained a reputation for being particularly helpful, working in tandem with the body's natural rhythms, offering a more harmonious approach to symptom management compared to conventional treatments that often come with a risk of side effects.

The beauty of these herbs is that they work with your body, not against it. They're like a friend who knows exactly what you're going through and has the right advice. Unlike some conventional treatments that can feel like they're bulldozing through your system with all sorts of side effects, these medicinal herbs are more like a gentle nudge in the right direction. They sync up with your body's natural rhythms, bringing a sense of harmony and balance that's often missing during this rollercoaster phase of life. The synergy between diet, nutrition, and medicinal herbs cannot be overstated. As we've emphasized the importance of incorporating phytoestrogen-rich foods and maintaining a balanced diet, integrating specific herbs can further enhance these nutritional efforts. Let's consider how incorporating herbs like red clover, and dong quai into our diet can provide a complementary boost, each herb bringing its unique properties to support our hormonal balance, emotional well-being, and overall health during menopause.

Red Clover

Red clover is like nature's own version of hormone therapy, but with a soft touch. Its claim to fame in the world of menopausal support comes from its rich composition of isoflavones. Isoflavones, plant based compounds, are a specific type of phytoestrogen predominantly found in soy and are known for their estrogen-like effects in the body, making them particularly relevant in discussions about natural treatments for menopause and other conditions related to estrogen levels. As we know by now, lots of menopause symptoms are caused by the fluctuation and gradual decline of estrogen levels in the body. This is where red clover steps in, offering a helping hand to balance things out.

Think of red clover as a kind of botanical hormone balancer. It's like having a subtle, natural ally in your corner, working quietly to ease some of those hallmark symptoms of menopause. Many women turn to red clover for relief from hot flashes, but the potential benefits of red clover extend far beyond. As our estrogen levels dip, our bones can become more vulnerable. Using red clover, with its plant-based phytoestrogens, is a great way to also fortify your bones against the ebbs and flows of hormonal change, something we'll talk a lot more on in Chapter 4.

Dong Quai

Dong quai, with its esteemed title as the 'female ginseng,' holds a special place in the world of medicinal herbs, particularly for women navigating the complexities of menopause. This herb, deeply rooted in traditional Chinese medicine, is believed to be a harmonizer of the body's systems, particularly focusing on women's health.

Dong quai's purported ability to balance hormones is what makes it a standout choice for us when experiencing menopausal symptoms. Dong quai is thought to help ease these transitions, providing a more natural, gentle approach to hormone regulation.

In traditional Chinese medicine, Dong quai is often used as a blood tonic. This means it's believed to help improve circulation and nourish the blood. Good circulation is crucial for overall health and can particularly benefit us menopausal women, facing potential changes in blood pressure or slower circulation. Improved blood flow can also contribute to better mental clarity and energy levels, countering some of the fatigue and brain fog that often accompany menopause.

Additionally, Dong quai is sometimes used for its potential to alleviate joint discomfort and muscle aches, symptoms that we might encounter during menopause. Its anti-inflammatory properties are believed to help in reducing pain and improving mobility. Compared to red clover, it's more of an all rounder.

Incorporating medicinal herbs like red clover, and dong quai into your daily life can be a practical and enjoyable part of managing menopause symptoms. Here's how you can integrate these herbs into your routine:

- Teas and Infusions: One of the simplest ways to enjoy these herbs is in tea form. Herbal teas made from red clover or dong quai can be consumed daily. You can find these teas at health food stores or online. Steep the tea as per instructions, usually for about 5-10 minutes. Start with one cup a day and see how your body responds.
- Incorporate into Meals: Red clover can be used in culinary preparations. Its sprouts can be added to salads, sandwiches, and other dishes for a subtle phytoestrogen boost.

Medicinal herbs often take time to show their full effects. Incorporate them into your daily routine for a consistent period (usually a few weeks to a couple of months) to properly evaluate their impact. It's also worth getting personalized advice and dosage recommendations; consider consulting with a herbalist or naturopath. They can tailor a regimen that suits your specific symptoms and overall health profile. And as always, pay attention to how your body responds. Herbs can interact with medications and other supplements, so it's crucial to monitor for any adverse reactions and consult with your healthcare provider.

PRACTICAL DIETARY ADJUSTMENTS FOR MENOPAUSE

Let's look at how you can tweak your intake of carbohydrates, proteins, and fats to better suit your body's changing needs during this time.

Making Smart Choices with Carbohydrates

Carbohydrates often get a bad rap, but they're an important energy source. The key is choosing carbs that release energy slowly, keeping you fueled and satisfied for longer.

Many of us can find ourselves with a 'lazy' keto diet that doesn't include enough fiber; this can contribute to more hormonal imbalance and sleep disruptions in menopause.

It is important to eat good quality carbs. These are your whole grains, like brown rice, quinoa, and whole-wheat pasta, as well as starchy vegetables like sweet potatoes. They're packed with fiber, which is great for digestion and can help manage blood sugar levels. Try swapping out white bread for whole-grain varieties or replacing white rice with quinoa in your next meal.

Prioritizing Quality Proteins

Protein is crucial for maintaining muscle mass, which naturally starts to decrease as we age. Including good quality protein in your diet is like adding building blocks to maintain your muscle strength. Typically a woman in the menopause transition needs 2 to 4 grams per kilogram of body weight per day depending on their level of activity, An easy way to think of that is a palm sized serving of protein at every meal.

Lean meats, poultry, fish, eggs, dairy, and plant-based sources like beans, lentils, and tofu are great options. How about starting your day with a Greek yogurt or adding some grilled chicken or chickpeas to your salads? Remember, it's not just about quantity; it's the quality of protein that counts.

Embracing Healthy Fats

Fats are essential, especially omega-3 fatty acids, which are heroes for hormone production and heart health and helping the body manage inflammation. Many women don't get enough Omega 3s, yet every cell in your body needs them - especially the eyes and brain. They are also important for muscle activity, immune function, digestion and fertility.

Risk of heart disease increases after menopause. Omega 3s may help keep triglyceride levels in check. They may also help with psychological issues, depression, and hot flashes.

It is recommended that women consume 1100 mg of omega-3s daily. These fats, found in fish like salmon and mackerel, as well as in firm tofu, flaxseeds, chia seeds, and walnuts, are like lubricants for your body, keeping everything running smoothly. Try to incorporate these into your meals regularly. It can be as simple as sprinkling some chia seeds on your breakfast cereal, enjoying a handful of walnuts as a snack, or baking a salmon filet for dinner. Supplementing with a high quality omega 3 oil can help to give you the required daily intake.

Remember, menopause is a unique experience for every woman. It's important to listen to your body and adjust your diet according to how you feel. If a certain food doesn't agree with you or if you find a particular macronutrient balance works better, trust that instinct. This period of your life is about embracing change and finding what keeps you feeling your best.

Adjusting your diet during menopause is about being mindful and responsive to your body's needs. By making these tweaks in your macronutrient intake and focusing on hormone-supportive foods, you're setting the stage for a healthier, more comfortable menopausal transition.

UNDERSTANDING AND TACKLING INFLAMMATION DURING MENOPAUSE

Inflammation is like your body's natural defense system, responding to injuries or invaders like bacteria. As estrogen, progesterone and testosterone decline during the menopause transition, inflammation in your body can rise. When this is coupled with unchecked stress aka high cortisol levels and a diet high in ultra processed foods, over time this systemic inflammation can damage our arteries, organs, and joints, increasing our risk for chronic disease like heart disease, arthritis, dementia, and other conditions.

Ways to counteract this inflammation begin by going easy on foods that contribute to inflammation in the body such as ultra-processed refined carbs, sugary beverages, processed meats, and fried foods. As well as managing stress and getting sufficient sleep.

Consider an anti-inflammatory diet, which is like choosing the right team to calm down that overactive defense system. It's genuinely amazing how much we can mitigate the difficult symptoms of menopause with the right 'diet toolbox'. Popular diets like the Mediterranean and MIND diets (the MIND Diet is a hybrid between the MedDiet and Dietary Approach to Stop Hypertension, or DASH Diet) are known for their anti-inflammatory properties.

Later in this chapter, we'll look at practical examples of how you can incorporate anti-inflammatory foods into your diet incrementally. For now, here's a lineup of some anti-inflammatory winners:

- Berries: These little gems are packed with antioxidants and vitamins. Blueberries, strawberries, and raspberries can be your go-to snacks or breakfast toppings.
- Leafy Greens: Vegetables like spinach, kale, and Swiss chard are rich in vitamins and low in calories. They're like natural warriors against inflammation.
- Nuts: Almonds, walnuts, and other nuts are not only great for snacking but also bring healthy fats and proteins to your anti-inflammatory arsenal.
- Fatty Fish: Salmon, mackerel, and sardines are rich in omega-3 fatty acids, which are excellent at reducing inflammation. They're like your body's peacekeepers, working to keep inflammation in check.

INTEGRATING NUTRITION WITH LIFESTYLE FOR HOLISTIC HEALTH

Hydration during menopause is like oil in an engine – it keeps everything running smoothly. Water plays a crucial role in almost every bodily function, and its importance only escalates during menopause. As we age our bodies don't retain as much water, when we are younger we are 70% water but by the time we get to menopause we may be only 55% water which is a substantial drop.

Adequate hydration can help manage symptoms like brain fog, dry skin, reduce the frequency of hot flashes, reduce urinary urgency, relieve headaches and muscle cramps and even aid in weight management. It's recommended to drink at least 8-10 glasses of water daily, but listen to your body – it might need more, especially if you're active or live in a hot climate. Remember, herbal teas and water-rich fruits and vegetables also count towards your fluid intake.

Finding the right balance between what you eat and how much you move is key to maintaining optimal health during menopause. It's like a dance – your diet provides the energy, and physical activity uses that energy in a beautiful rhythm. If you're more active, you might need more calories or certain nutrients. Conversely, if your lifestyle is more sedentary, your dietary needs may differ.

Regular physical activity helps in managing weight, improving mood, and maintaining muscle mass. Align your diet to support your activity level – a little extra protein on workout days, or some healthy carbs for energy. It's about creating a harmony between your diet and your physical activity to feel your best.

THE GUT MICROBIOME

You might be wondering, how does gut health tie in here, and how does it affect things such as hormone regulation during menopause? Well, it's a two-way street. The health of our gut can influence the balance and regulation of hormones, and these hormonal changes can, in turn, impact our gut health. It's a delicate dance of mutual influence.

Now, let's talk about those tiny yet powerful inhabitants of our gut – microorganisms. These microscopic beings are not just passive dwellers; they actively participate in metabolizing estrogens. This is particularly important during menopause when estrogen levels fluctuate. An imbalance in our gut flora can lead to less efficient estrogen metabolism, which can then exacerbate common menopausal symptoms like hot flashes and mood swings. It's like a ripple effect, where the state of our gut can have far-reaching impacts on our menopausal experience.

Here's the interesting part: the gut microbes are instrumental in breaking down and recycling hormones, particularly estrogen. This process is crucial for maintaining hormonal balance. However, during menopause, as estrogen levels fluctuate and eventually decline, this can impact the gut environment. Changes in estrogen levels can affect gut motility, leading to issues like constipation or diarrhea. It's a bit like a dance, where one partner's move influences the other's.

Conversely, the health of your gut also impacts hormone regulation. A healthy gut with a balanced microbiome aids in efficient hormone metabolism. But if your gut health is compromised – say, by an imbalance in gut flora or poor diet – it can lead to inefficient estrogen metabolism. This inefficiency can exacerbate menopausal symptoms, such as hot flashes or mood swings. Think of it as a feedback loop where gut health and hormone regulation continuously influence each other.

Recent years have seen a burgeoning interest in the gut-hormone connection, particularly regarding its impact on menopausal health. Studies have begun to unravel how this intricate relationship influences the severity and management of menopause symptoms. One landmark study in the field, as outlined by the *Journal of Endocrinological Investigation*, investigates the role of the gut microbiome in estrogen metabolism. The research highlights how certain strains of gut bacteria, known as the estrobolome, are responsible for metabolizing estrogen. This process is pivotal for maintaining hormonal balance within the body. The findings suggest that disruptions in the gut microbiome can lead to imbalances in estrogen levels, potentially exacerbating menopausal symptoms such as hot flashes, mood swings, and osteoporosis.

Another significant piece of research, published in *Menopause*, the journal of The North American Menopause Society, delves into the effects of probiotic supplementation on menopausal women. The research team conducted a randomized, double-blind, placebo-controlled trial involving a group of menopausal women who were not undergoing any form of hormone replacement therapy. Participants were divided into two groups: one received a daily probiotic supplement containing strains known to impact the gut-estrogen axis positively, while the control group received a placebo.

Over the course of several months, the study observed notable differences between the two groups. Women who took the probiotic supplement reported a significant reduction in the frequency and severity of hot flashes, one of the most common and disruptive symptoms of menopause. Additionally, improvements were noted in vaginal health, with participants experiencing less dryness and discomfort, which are indicative of a healthier vaginal microbiome.

The probiotic group also reported enhanced mood stability and reduced instances of menopause-related depression and anxiety. These mood improvements suggest a potential link between gut health and the regulation of stress hormones and neurotransmitters that influence mood.

Let's break down what this study on probiotics and menopause means for you in plain English, shall we? Imagine your gut as a bustling city where the right balance of residents (in this case, bacteria) makes everything run smoothly. During menopause, it's like the city is undergoing a massive overhaul - things get a bit chaotic, to say the least. This study suggests that bringing in some friendly new residents (probiotics) can help calm the chaos, making life in the city (your body) a bit more manageable. Ultimately the findings here were that women who added these probiotic superheroes to their daily routine noticed fewer hot flashes, less of that annoying vaginal dryness, and even saw their moods level out. It's not a magic potion, but it's a simple, natural way to potentially ease some of those pesky menopausal symptoms.

PREBIOTICS: THE ESSENTIAL NOURISHMENT FOR YOUR GUT'S BENEFICIAL BACTERIA

In the vast city of our gut microbiome, prebiotics play the crucial role of nourishment for probiotics, the beneficial bacteria that navigate the many streets of our digestive system. These prebiotics are found in a variety of foods, including garlic, onions, and asparagus, and are composed mainly of non-digestible fiber compounds. When we consume these foods, we're not digesting these fibers ourselves. Instead, they pass through the upper part of our gastrointestinal tract undigested and serve as food for the beneficial bacteria in our lower gut.

The relationship between prebiotics and probiotics is a symbiotic one, where the success of one directly benefits the other. Prebiotics are essentially the fuel that feeds our probiotic bacteria, allowing them to multiply, thrive, and perform their crucial functions. This includes everything from aiding digestion to synthesizing essential nutrients and bolstering our immune system. By ensuring a steady supply of prebiotics through our diet, we support a thriving community of probiotics in our gut, which is essential for maintaining overall health and particularly beneficial during the hormonal fluctuations of menopause. Soluble fibers, found in foods like oats, nuts, seeds, and some fruits and vegetables, are particularly effective as prebiotics.

Dietary fiber serves multiple functions in our digestive system, one of which is acting as a prebiotic. However, not all fibers are created equal. There are soluble fibers, which dissolve in water and can help to soften our stools, making them easier to pass. Then there are insoluble fibers, which do not dissolve in water and add bulk to our stool, helping prevent constipation. Both types of fiber are important for digestive health, but they also play distinct roles in nurturing our gut microbiome. Insoluble fibers, found in whole grains, wheat bran, and vegetables, help to move waste through the digestive system and can help prevent the buildup of harmful bacteria.

A diverse, fiber-rich diet ensures that you're providing a broad spectrum of prebiotics to feed various beneficial microbes in your gut. This diversity is key because just as our body needs a wide range of nutrients to function optimally, our gut microbiome thrives on a varied diet to maintain its health and diversity. This is particularly important during menopause, a time when hormonal changes can disrupt gut health, leading to symptoms like bloating, constipation, or even exacerbating mood swings and hot flashes. By focusing on a diet rich in prebiotics and fiber, you're doing so much more than just feeding your body; you're cultivating a gut environment that can better withstand the hormonal shifts of menopause, supporting your overall health and well-being during this transition.

THE GUT-BRAIN CONNECTION

Perhaps one of the most fascinating aspects of gut health is its connection to the brain, known as the gut-brain axis. Diving deeper into the gut-brain connection unveils a remarkable insight into how our bodies and minds are intricately linked, especially during menopause. The gut-brain axis facilitates a two-way communication between the central nervous system and the gastrointestinal tract. It's a complex network that not only regulates digestion but also has a profound impact on our emotional and mental well-being.

Imagine your gut as a second brain, one that speaks directly to your mind, influencing feelings and thoughts. This isn't just poetic metaphor; it's grounded in scientific reality. The gut is home to an extensive network of neurons and is the primary source of serotonin production within the body. Serotonin is often associated with feelings of happiness and well-being. Its production in the gut means that the state of your digestive system can directly affect your mood. During menopause, when emotional roller coasters become more common due to hormonal fluctuations, having a well-balanced gut microbiome could be your secret weapon in maintaining emotional equilibrium.

But how does gut health actually influence mood swings and cognitive clarity during menopause? It's all about the chemicals and hormones produced and regulated within the gut. These substances can signal the brain to adjust mood, stress levels, and even pain perception. For instance, a diverse and thriving gut microbiome facilitates the production of serotonin, which then travels to the brain to promote feelings of happiness and reduce stress (and as we know, improved sleep!). Conversely, an imbalance in gut bacteria can lead to reduced serotonin levels, contributing to feelings of depression or anxiety.

Moreover, the gut-brain axis plays a role in managing stress responses. The adrenal glands, which are pivotal in the body's stress response, are influenced by signals from both the brain and the gut. A healthy gut can help moderate the body's reaction to stress, making you more resilient to the emotional upheavals that menopause can bring. In essence, nurturing your gut health is akin to nurturing your mental health! It's clear that gut health is not just a footnote in the story of menopause; it's a central character.

PRACTICAL TIPS FOR DAILY DIETS THAT PROMOTE A HEALTHY GUT, HORMONAL BALANCE & ANTI-INFLAMMATION

Tying everything together - our discussions on holistic therapies, inflammation, and the vital role of diet in managing menopause - it's clear that what we eat significantly impacts our journey through this transition. When it comes to meal planning, think about balance and variety. Plan your meals around these anti-inflammatory foods, mixing and matching them throughout the week. A good tip is to prepare some of these ingredients in advance – like washing and chopping your veggies or pre-cooking a batch of quinoa – so putting together a healthy, inflammation-fighting meal becomes a breeze. Integrating prebiotics and a diverse, fiber-rich diet is a massive part of this too for a healthy gut. Here's how you can seamlessly incorporate these elements into your daily routine:

- **Breakfast:** Let's revisit the concept of starting your day on the right note. A bowl of yogurt or kefir is a foundation for introducing beneficial probiotics into your gut. Enhance this with a sprinkle of flaxseed - not only for its prebiotic properties but also as a source of omega-3 fatty acids, which we've discussed as essential for hormonal balance and reducing inflammation. You could also start your day with a berry smoothie or oatmeal topped with a handful of nuts and fresh berries for an anti-inflammatory boost. This combination sets a positive tone for your digestive system, supporting gut health from the moment you begin your day and keeping inflammation at bay.
- **Lunch:** Remember the importance of incorporating varied, colorful foods into your meals to support overall well-being? A side of sauerkraut with your lunch or a salad dressed with raw onions and garlic isn't just a way to add flavor; it's a strategic move to feed your gut's beneficial bacteria. These foods, rich in prebiotics, encourage a healthy microbiome, which is crucial for metabolizing estrogens and maintaining hormonal equilibrium during menopause. A leafy green salad with grilled salmon or a kale and quinoa bowl can be a perfect anti-inflammatory midday meal.
- **Dinner:** Asparagus, with its high fiber content and prebiotic benefits, makes an excellent side dish for dinner. A side of steamed greens goes with anything

and has great anti-inflammatory benefits Alternatively, incorporating beans into your meals not only provides a fiber-rich punch but also contributes plant-based protein, aligning with our recommendations for a balanced diet that supports hormonal health.
- **Snacks:** We've touched on the value of fermented foods beyond just their taste. Snacking on pickles or a small serving of kimchi introduces additional probiotics into your diet, promoting gut health. Remember, maintaining a healthy gut microbiome is linked to reduced menopause symptoms, from hot flashes to mood swings, making these snacks more than just a midday treat. By making these small, intentional choices throughout your day, you're not just feeding your body; you're nurturing your well-being through menopause. This all feeds back into the holistic perspective we're embracing throughout this book, where every meal and every food choice plays a part in a larger strategy for your health and happiness during menopause!

When it comes to diet during menopause, one size does not fit all. Each body is unique, and so are its nutritional needs. It's important to consider your own health conditions, food preferences, and lifestyle when designing your diet. For example, if you have a specific condition like diabetes or heart disease, your dietary needs will be different. Listen to your body and how it responds to different foods. Some might find dairy doesn't suit them anymore, while others might thrive on a plant-based diet. An obvious one here given how much I've praised nuts as an all-encompassing antidote food to menopause symptoms, is if you're allergic to nuts then it might make sense to reap those same benefits from more emphasis on the greens and fatty fish oils. It's also worth considering consulting with a nutritionist or a healthcare provider who can help tailor your diet to your individual needs.

Consistency is key. It's not about being perfect every day; it's about making healthier choices most of the time. It's not about jumping on the latest diet fad; it's about making sustainable changes that you can stick with long term. Start with small, manageable changes, like incorporating more fruits and vegetables into your meals, choosing whole grains over refined ones, or reducing your sugar intake. Over time, these small changes can lead to significant, lasting impacts on your health and well-being. And remember, it's okay to treat yourself occasionally. A sustainable diet is flexible and adaptable – it's about balance, not deprivation.

CONCLUSION

Your dietary choices during menopause are not merely about sustenance; they're about making conscious decisions that honor your body's evolving requirements. Integrating nutrition with your lifestyle means acknowledging and responding to these changes with mindfulness and intention. It's about finding joy in the foods that bring comfort, energy, and balance, and allowing your diet to be a dynamic, responsive part of your life's tapestry. This adaptability in your approach to eating ensures that as you navigate through menopause, you do so with a sense of fulfillment and contentment.

Chapter Takeaways:

- Incorporating phytoestrogen-rich foods like soy, flaxseeds, and certain nuts can help balance hormonal shifts naturally.
- Essential nutrients such as calcium, vitamin D, magnesium, and the B vitamins are crucial for bone health, energy production, and mood regulation during menopause.
- A healthy gut microbiome supports hormone regulation, reduces menopause symptoms, and enhances mental well-being through the gut-brain connection.
- Herbs like red clover, and dong quai offer natural support for managing menopause symptoms, working in harmony with your body.
- An anti-inflammatory diet, rich in berries, leafy greens, and omega-3 fatty acids, can help mitigate the systemic inflammation often associated with menopause.
- Balancing diet with regular physical activity, stress management, and adequate hydration is essential for comprehensive menopausal well-being.
- Customizing your diet to your unique needs and being responsive to how different foods affect you is key to finding what works best for you during menopause.

Recommended listening for this chapter, from the Thriving Thru Menopause Podcast:

- Season 2 Episode 48: The Natural Menopause
- Season 6 Episode 2. How to Fire Up Your Metabolism in Menopause
- Season 5 Episode 16: The Gut Microbiome and its role in menopause
- Season 3 Episode 21: A Gutsy Menopause

Scan This QR Code To Listen On Your Favorite Podcast App

PHYSICAL ACTIVITY & EXERCISE

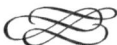

*L*et's talk about physical activity in managing the unique challenges of menopause. In this chapter, you'll discover how exercise is not just about maintaining fitness; it's a vital key to alleviating common menopausal symptoms, enhancing mood, and safeguarding your long-term health. From understanding the role of endorphins in mood regulation to customizing an exercise routine that resonates with your lifestyle, this chapter is a roadmap to embracing an active life during menopause. Get ready to explore how the right blend of physical activities can be your ally in navigating this significant life transition with grace and vitality.

THE POWER OF EXERCISE IN EASING MENOPAUSE SYMPTOMS

As you navigate the ups and downs of menopause, regular exercise can be a vital anchor, providing stability and relief from some of the most common menopausal symptoms.

Let's explore how staying active can be a game-changer during this phase of your life.

Hot flashes, mood swings, and weight gain might just well be the notorious trio of menopause. But here's the good news: regular exercise can help manage all three.

- Cooling Down Hot Flashes: Think of exercise as your personal thermostat. While the science behind it is still evolving, many women report a reduction in the frequency and intensity of hot flashes with regular physical activity. It's like giving your body a natural cooling system.
- Smoothing Out Mood Swings: Exercise is like an emotional balancer. It's not just about the physical benefits; it's also about giving your mental health a boost. Engaging in physical activity can help even out those mood swings, bringing a sense of calm and stability to your day.
- Managing Weight Gain: As metabolism changes during menopause, maintaining a healthy weight can become more challenging. Regular exercise importantly helps to maintain and build muscle, which in turn helps to boost your metabolism. It's like hitting multiple birds with one stone – you manage your weight while improving overall health.

You might already be linking together how the combination of intentional nutrition that we discussed in the last chapter with regular exercise, can be a superpower during menopause!

THE JOY OF ENDORPHINS

Physical activity is a natural mood lifter. When you exercise, your body releases endorphins, those feel-good chemicals that boost your mood and bring a sense of well-being. It's like your body's natural antidepressant. Whether it's a brisk walk or a yoga session, you're not just working out your body; you're giving your mind a dose of happiness.

When you exercise, especially during activities that raise your heart rate, your body recognizes this as a form of stress. In response, it increases endorphin production to help ease this stress. It's like your body's own way of saying, "It's okay, I've got this." This endorphin rush is often referred to as the 'runner's high,' but you don't have to be a runner to experience it. Any form of moderate to vigorous physical activity can trigger this delightful release. This release through exercise can be particularly beneficial during menopause, a time often marked by mood swings, depression, or anxiety. These endorphins can help lift your mood, reduce feelings of depression, and decrease anxiety levels. It's like a natural antidote to the emotional rollercoaster of menopause.

Let's face it though, there will be days during menopause when the last thing you feel like doing is exercising. Maybe you're feeling low, tired, or just out of sorts. But here's a little secret – those are the days when exercise can actually help the most.

Think of physical activity as a gentle nudge to your mood. On days when you're not feeling up to it, the key is to start small. Instead of aiming for an intense workout, go for a brief walk around the block or a short stretching session. Often, the hardest part is just getting started. Once you're moving, those endorphins begin to flow, and you might just find your mood lifting almost without you realizing it.

For those times when life gets hectic and it feels like there's no room for exercise, remember that every little bit counts. It's not about carving out huge chunks of time; it's about finding small opportunities throughout your day. This could be a quick 10-minute walk, a few minutes of stretching in the morning, or some light yoga before bed. These small sessions can add up and are better than no activity at all. Another way is to get creative with your routines. Dance while you're cooking, do calf raises while brushing your teeth, or take the stairs instead of the elevator! It's about making movement a natural part of your day.

And as is a running theme here throughout this book (and menopause itself), always listen to your body. Some days you might be up for more, and other days less – and that's perfectly okay. Menopause is a time of change, and being flexible with your exercise routine is key. It's about finding a balance that works for you, where exercise is a source of joy and rejuvenation, not a chore.

The beauty of exercise is that it's not one-size-fits-all. Whether you're a seasoned athlete or just starting out, there's an activity for you.

- Walking: Simple yet effective. It's a great way to start if you're new to exercise. All you need is a pair of comfortable shoes, and you're set.

- Swimming: Perfect for those looking for a low-impact option. It's easy on the joints and can be quite soothing.
- Yoga: Combines physical postures with breathing exercises. It's great for flexibility, balance, and stress relief.
- Pilates: whether mat exercises or reformer machines can help develop a good posture to support your joints, improve flexibility and balance. It can strengthen the core muscles weakened by menopause.

Remember, the best exercise is the one you enjoy and can stick with. It's all about finding what works for you and making it a regular part of your routine.

MIND-BODY PRACTICES

Mind-body practices like yoga, tai chi, and meditation are a huge part of the picture when looking to manage menopause holistically. Bringing huge benefits in the realms of both physical exercise and mental clarity and calmness, mind-body practices are an embodiment of what it means to take a holistic approach to menopause.

Today, these things can feel almost overdone, with them trending everywhere and being recommended to basically anyone. Navigating through menopause, you might wonder, "Will these mind-body practices truly work for me?" It's a valid question. After all, menopause is not just another phase; it's a profound shift, and each of us experiences it uniquely. But that's precisely where the beauty of yoga, tai chi, and meditation lies – their flexibility and adaptability to our individual needs and experiences.

When faced with the diverse options of yoga, tai chi, and meditation for stress relief and exercise during menopause, you might feel a bit overwhelmed. "Which one should I choose?" you might ask. The answer lies in personalization and experimentation. Menopause is as individual as you are, and the key is to find what resonates with your body, mind, and lifestyle.

Start by assessing your current needs and preferences. If you're looking for a practice that combines gentle physical activity with stress reduction, yoga might be your best bet. It offers the dual benefit of soothing your body while calming your mind. On days when you feel physically drained but still want to engage in a mindful practice, yoga can be adapted to be less about challenging poses and more about gentle stretches and breathing. There are various styles and poses, each offering different benefits. If hot flashes or night sweats are your main concern, certain cooling and restorative yoga poses can be particularly beneficial. These poses are designed to soothe the nervous system and help regulate body temperature. And if it's the mood swings or irritability that trouble you the most, yoga's focus on breathwork and mindfulness can be incredibly grounding.

If the idea of meditative movement appeals to you, tai chi could be the perfect fit. Its slow, flowing movements are ideal for those who might find sitting still in meditation challenging, and of course this way of doing it means more in the way of exercise too. Tai chi is particularly beneficial if you're looking for a practice that enhances balance and coordination, which can sometimes be affected during menopause. For many women in menopause, tai chi can also be a gateway to better stress management and emotional regulation.

And if racing thoughts or anxiety is what's top of mind for you, meditation could be the answer. The thought of sitting still with your thoughts might be daunting, especially if your mind is constantly racing with menopausal anxieties. But that's exactly why meditation can be so powerful. It teaches you to observe your thoughts without getting swept away by them - a skill that can be particularly helpful during menopause when your emotions might feel more volatile. Meditation doesn't require you to clear your mind; it's about learning to find peace amidst the mental chatter. Finding stillness in the chaos and learning to observe your thoughts without getting lost in them.

This might seem like a lot of options, and you might be wondering where to even begin. Give yourself permission to explore and experiment. Try a yoga class one week, a tai chi session the next, and incorporate short meditations into your daily routine, 10 minute guided YouTube videos are a perfect place to start. Pay attention to how each practice makes you feel. Which one leaves you feeling more balanced, more at peace, or more energized? That's the compass you should follow. Your menopause journey is uniquely yours, and the path you choose for stress relief should be just as personalized. Trust your instincts - they are your best guide in this phase of life. The aim isn't to do all of these, but to try them out and find what's right for you. I gave the selection of these 3 practices in particular as combined, they cover all grounds when it comes to a holistic solution to menopause, so by giving them all a try, you'll almost certainly find that one of them in particular will suit you perfectly.

DEVELOPING A PERSONALIZED EXERCISE PLAN FOR MENOPAUSE

Embarking on an exercise journey during menopause starts with understanding where you are right now. It's like plotting your starting point on a map before you set off on a journey. To assess your current fitness level, consider a few simple questions: How often do you currently exercise? What types of activities do you engage in, and for how long? How do you feel during and after exercising – energized, exhausted, or somewhere in between?

Also, think about your recent health history. Have you had any injuries or conditions that might affect your ability to exercise? Understanding your starting point helps in setting realistic and achievable goals. It's about challenging yourself without pushing too hard, to avoid injury and burnout.

A well-rounded exercise routine is like a balanced diet – it should include a mix of different types of activities. Variety not only keeps things interesting but also ensures a comprehensive approach to your fitness.

- Cardiovascular Exercises: These are exercises that get your heart rate up, like brisk walking, jogging, swimming, or cycling. They're great for heart health and stamina.
- Strength Training: This includes activities that build muscle strength, such as using weights, resistance bands, or body-weight exercises like squats and

push-ups. Strength training is crucial for bone health and managing weight.
- Flexibility Exercises: Practices like yoga or pilates are great for maintaining mobility and preventing injury.

By incorporating a mix of these exercises, you're not just working on different aspects of your physical health; you're also keeping your workouts engaging and fun.

Menopause can bring days of high energy and days when you might not feel like moving at all. Listen to your body and adapt your exercise routine accordingly. On days when you feel full of energy, you might engage in more vigorous activities. On lower-energy days, something gentler like a walk or a yoga session might be more appropriate.

It's also important to pay attention to how your body responds to exercise during menopause. You might find that you need more time to recover, or certain exercises don't feel as comfortable as they used to. Don't hesitate to modify exercises to fit your comfort level.

Remember, exercising during menopause is not about sticking rigidly to a plan; it's about flexibility and adaptation. It's perfectly okay to adjust your activities based on how you feel each day. The goal is to stay active in a way that supports your body and your menopause journey.

THE ROLE OF EXERCISE IN BONE HEALTH AND CARDIOVASCULAR FITNESS

During menopause, the decrease in estrogen can lead to a decrease in bone density, raising the risk of osteoporosis. Imagine your bones as a bank account where you make 'bone deposits' and 'withdrawals' throughout your life. After menopause, it's crucial to keep making deposits to maintain bone strength.

But firstly, what could constitute a 'bone withdrawal?' These are factors or activities that can potentially weaken your bones or decrease bone density over time. Just like a financial withdrawal reduces your bank balance, bone withdrawals can diminish the strength and health of your bones. Here are some common examples:

- Lack of Physical Activity: Leading a sedentary lifestyle is one of the biggest bone withdrawals. Without regular exercise, especially weight-bearing and muscle-strengthening activities, bones can lose their density and strength, becoming more prone to fractures.
- Poor Nutrition: Not getting enough calcium and vitamin D is like making continuous withdrawals from your bone bank. These nutrients are crucial for bone health, and a deficiency can lead to weaker bones. Similarly, excessive intake of salt, caffeine, or alcohol can also negatively impact bone density.
- Smoking: Smoking is known to have a detrimental effect on bone health. It interferes with the body's

ability to absorb calcium, leading to weaker bones and increasing the risk of osteoporosis.
- Certain Medications: Some medications, when used long-term, can lead to bone loss. For example, corticosteroids and some anticonvulsants are known to affect bone density.
- Hormonal Changes in Menopause: The decline in estrogen during menopause is a significant factor in bone density loss. Estrogen plays a vital role in maintaining bone health, and its reduction can accelerate bone density loss.
- Excessive Stress: Chronic stress can lead to hormonal imbalances that negatively impact bone health. Stress hormones can interfere with the body's ability to rebuild and maintain strong bones.

Understanding these 'bone withdrawals' is crucial in menopause. It highlights the importance of counteracting these factors through lifestyle choices like regular exercise, a balanced diet rich in bone-healthy nutrients, quitting smoking, and managing stress. By being aware of these factors and actively working to minimize their impact, you can help maintain strong, healthy bones throughout menopause and beyond.

Okay, so how do we regularly deposit into our 'bone health balance?' Weight-bearing exercises, like walking, jogging, tennis, and dancing, force you to work against gravity. They're like making regular deposits into your bone health bank. Resistance exercises, such as lifting weights or using resistance bands, are equally important. They're like giving your bones a healthy challenge, encouraging them to maintain their strength.

By integrating these types of exercises into your routine, you're not just working out; you're actively fighting against the risk of osteoporosis and keeping your bones robust and resilient. Remember that Exercises also help to protect against falls. Osteoporosis is associated with an increased risk of falls that incur fracture,

IMPROVING HEART HEALTH: PROTECTING YOUR LIFELINE

Heart disease is the number one killer of women worldwide and the risk of developing it tends to increase after menopause, making cardiovascular health more important than ever. Regular physical activity is like a guardian for your heart. It helps in managing weight, reducing blood pressure, and lowering bad cholesterol levels, all of which are crucial for maintaining a healthy heart.

It's recommended that women accumulate at least 150 minutes per week of moderate exercise (such as brisk walking) or 75 minutes per week of vigorous exercise. The activity can be spread throughout the week in at least 10-minute sessions. Resistance training is also recommended for 20 minute sessions, two to three times a week. Think of these activities as giving your heart the workout it needs to stay fit and strong. By regularly engaging in these exercises, you're not only enhancing your heart's health but also improving your overall endurance and vitality.

Menopause doesn't just mark a hormonal shift; it can also signal a change in how your body processes and manages energy. This phase can sometimes tip the scales towards metabolic syndrome, a group of conditions that raise the risk of heart disease, stroke, and type 2 diabetes. Think of your metabolism as an engine. During menopause, this engine can start to work less efficiently, leading to high blood pressure, elevated blood sugar levels, unwanted weight gain (especially around the abdomen), and abnormal cholesterol levels.

HOW REGULAR EXERCISE REJUVENATES YOUR METABOLIC ENGINE

Regular exercise is like a tune-up for your metabolic engine, ensuring it runs smoothly and efficiently. Here's how it helps:

- Regulating Blood Sugar: Physical activity helps in controlling insulin sensitivity. When you exercise, your muscles use up glucose for energy, which in turn helps in lowering blood sugar levels. Activities like brisk walking, swimming, or cycling are particularly beneficial in this regard.
- Maintaining Healthy Weight: Exercise, especially aerobic activities, burns calories and helps in managing weight. This is crucial because excess weight, particularly around the waist, is a key factor in metabolic syndrome.
- Reducing Abdominal Fat: Abdominal fat is more than just a cosmetic concern. It's closely linked with various metabolic disorders. Regular exercise helps

in targeting this visceral fat, reducing its accumulation.
- Boosting Muscle Mass: Strength training exercises, such as lifting weights or bodyweight exercises like push-ups and squats, build muscle mass. More muscle mass means a higher resting metabolic rate, meaning you burn more calories even when you're not actively exercising.

The best approach to exercise for metabolic health during menopause is a balanced one. Combine aerobic exercises (like jogging, cycling, or swimming) with strength training. This combination not only helps in burning calories but also in building and maintaining muscle mass, both of which are key for a healthy metabolism.

However, remember that consistency is more critical than intensity. Aim for moderate-intensity activities that you can incorporate regularly into your routine. It doesn't have to be long, grueling workouts. Even 30 minutes a day can make a significant difference. The goal is to find activities you enjoy, so it becomes a sustainable part of your lifestyle, not a chore.

CONCLUSION

We now know how crucial exercise becomes during menopause, transforming from just a way to stay fit into a lifeline for managing those pesky symptoms, boosting your mood, and securing your health for the future. This part of the book was all about showing you how to navigate menopause with energy and a smile, encouraging you to mix it up with everything from the soothing rhythms of yoga to empowering weight training sessions. Not to mention the mood-lifting magic of endorphins and the often forgotten sheer joy of movement! It was an invitation to find that perfect blend of physical activities that just click with your personal menopause journey, making this significant phase not just bearable but vibrant and full of life.

Chapter Takeaways:

- Regular physical activity can reduce hot flashes, stabilize mood swings, and counteract weight gain.
- Engaging in exercise releases endorphins, combating depression and anxiety, and fostering an overall sense of well-being.
- Tailoring your exercise regimen to fit your lifestyle and preferences ensures that physical activity remains a source of joy, not a chore. Don't forget to stay flexible with it and allow for adjustments based on energy levels and comfort.
- Incorporating yoga, tai chi, and meditation into your routine can enhance both physical health and mental clarity.
- Weight-bearing and resistance training exercises are pivotal in maintaining bone density and preventing osteoporosis.
- Regular exercise plays a key role in protecting heart health, which becomes even more crucial after menopause.
- A balanced mix of aerobic and strength training exercises can rejuvenate your metabolism, helping to manage weight and reduce the risk of metabolic syndrome.

Recommended listening for this chapter, from the Thriving Thru Menopause Podcast:

- Season 3 Episode 9: Strong, Active and Healthy
- Season 3 Episode 6: Fitness in Menopause
- Season 6 Episode 9 The Ultimate Guide to Staying Fit and Agile Over 50

Scan This QR Code To Listen On Your Favorite Podcast App

SLEEP MANAGEMENT

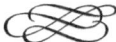

This chapter delves into the complex relationship between hormonal changes and sleep patterns, offering insight into how fluctuating and declining levels of estrogen and progesterone can significantly impact your sleep quality. We also explore other contributing factors like stress, lifestyle habits, and health conditions that can exacerbate sleep issues. By recognizing the symptoms and understanding their causes, this chapter empowers you to take control of your sleep, enhancing your overall well-being during this transitional phase.

According to the recent Evernow survey of 100K women, sleep disruption is the second most common symptom that affects 80% of women through perimenopause and menopause. It is often one the first symptoms of perimenopause and rated as the most debilitating symptoms of menopause. Poor sleep can exacerbate other symptoms including fatigue, brain fog and mood swings.

As you transition into menopause, understanding the changes in sleep patterns becomes crucial. It's not just about feeling rested; it's about comprehending the shifts occurring in your body, especially in your brain's sleep regulation mechanisms.

YOUR BRAIN AND SLEEP

The brain has specific areas and neurotransmitters responsible for promoting wakefulness and sleep. These areas work in a sort of balance, ensuring that you are either awake or asleep. Two primary factors regulate this balance: the sleep need (or sleep drive) and the biological clock.

- Sleep Need: This is straightforward. When you wake up, assuming a good night's sleep, your need for sleep is at its lowest. However, as the day progresses, this need gradually builds up, peaking in the evening when you feel ready to sleep.
- Biological Clock: This internal clock, located in your brain, sets the rhythm for all body processes, including sleep. It responds to external light cues to synchronize your body's functions with the day-night cycle. Light exposure, particularly in the morning, resets this clock daily.

HORMONES AND SLEEP: A MATTER OF BALANCE

By this point, we know that when you enter menopause, your body undergoes significant changes in estrogen and progesterone levels. It's less known that both play a crucial role in regulating sleep. Estrogen helps regulate the sleep-wake cycle, influences the production of serotonin (which in turn affects sleep), and contributes to the quality of REM (Rapid Eye Movement) sleep, which is crucial for cognitive functions like memory and learning.

Progesterone, often termed a 'sleep-promoting' hormone, enhances the quality of sleep by acting as a natural sedative. It also plays a role in breathing regulation during sleep. As these hormone levels decline, you might find yourself tossing and turning at night. This disruption can lead to common sleep issues like insomnia and frequent awakenings, often accompanied by night sweats.

These common sleep issues include:

- Difficulty Falling Asleep: Spending long hours trying to drift off.
- Trouble Staying Asleep: Waking up frequently during the night.
- Unrefreshing Sleep: Feeling tired even after a full night's sleep. This can often lead to fatigue and drowsiness during the day, impacting your overall energy levels and mood.

However, it's not just hormonal changes at play. Several other factors can exacerbate sleep disturbances during menopause:

- Stress and Anxiety: The menopausal transition can be a stressful time, and stress is a well-known enemy of good sleep. Anxiety about changes happening in your body can also keep your mind active at night.

- Lifestyle Habits: Certain habits like late-night caffeine intake, irregular sleep schedules, and excessive screen time before bed can further disrupt sleep.
- Other Health Conditions: Conditions common in menopausal women, such as sleep apnea, pain in the back or joints or restless leg syndrome, can also interfere with your sleep quality. An over or underactive thyroid can lead to sleep problems. Thyroid disorders are ten times more common in women than in men. The risk of developing an underactive thyroid also increases with age. If you suspect you are having problems it is important to discuss this with your healthcare provider.

During menopause, increased anxiety is a common experience that can significantly disrupt sleep. This heightened state of anxiety can be likened to a meerkat on high alert. Just as a meerkat stands guard, constantly scanning its environment for danger, menopausal women may find themselves in a similar state of hyper-alertness during the night. This can manifest as an overly sensitive response to environmental or internal changes, making it difficult to achieve deep, restful sleep.

The analogy of the meerkat helps to illustrate how this heightened state of vigilance, while a natural protective mechanism, can become counterproductive when it comes to sleep. In this state, the mind and body are constantly on edge, ready to react to any perceived threat, no matter how small. This can lead to a vicious cycle of sleep disturbances, where the fear or anxiety of not being able to sleep actually becomes the very thing that keeps you awake.

Managing this anxiety and stress is crucial for better sleep. The menopause guidelines in many countries recommend cognitive behavioral therapy CBT for sleep issues. It is also known that techniques such as mindfulness, relaxation exercises, can be effective in reducing stress and breaking the anxiety cycle.

By learning to acknowledge and then gently shift away from these anxious thoughts, you can help your body to relax and prepare for sleep. This process of 'coming off guard,' much like the meerkat eventually relaxing and returning to its normal activities, allows your body to move out of the hyper-alert state and into a more restful and sleep-conducive mode.

THE RELATIONSHIP BETWEEN SLEEP, HEALTH, AND MENOPAUSE SYMPTOMS

Poor sleep during menopause is not just an inconvenience; it can profound implications for long term health::

- Weight Gain: Hormonal changes in menopause can slow down metabolism, and when coupled with poor sleep, the propensity for weight gain increases. Lack of sleep can disrupt the balance of hunger hormones, leading to increased appetite and cravings for high-calorie, sugary foods.
- Diabetes Risk: Consistent lack of sleep affects the body's ability to use insulin effectively, increasing the risk of insulin resistance and type 2 diabetes. This is

particularly concerning during menopause, as changes in hormone levels already predispose women to a higher risk of diabetes.
- Heart Disease: Sleep disturbances have been linked to cardiovascular problems, including high blood pressure and heart disease. Poor sleep can lead to changes in the body that promote inflammation and stress, both of which are risk factors for heart conditions.
- Weakened Immune System: Sleep is crucial for the proper functioning of the immune system. Chronic sleep deprivation can weaken immune defenses, making you more susceptible to infections and potentially impacting the body's response to vaccines.

EFFECT ON MENTAL AND EMOTIONAL WELL-BEING

The impact of poor sleep on mental and emotional health during menopause is profound and multifaceted:

- Heightened Stress Levels: Lack of sleep can exacerbate the body's stress response, leading to increased production of cortisol, the stress hormone. This can create a vicious cycle where stress leads to poor sleep, which in turn leads to more stress.
- Mood Swings and Emotional Instability: Sleep deprivation affects the regulation of mood-related chemicals in the brain, leading to heightened emotional reactions and mood swings. This can

make the emotional roller coaster of menopause even more pronounced.
- Increased Risk of Depression and Anxiety: There's a strong link between sleep problems and mental health issues, including depression and anxiety. Insufficient sleep can amplify feelings of sadness, hopelessness, and worry, further complicating the menopause transition.

WAYS TO PROMOTE BETTER SLEEP

The Circadian Rhythm– Look on the Light Side

In the realm of improving sleep during menopause, the role of morning light exposure is crucial in regulating our internal biological clock, also known as the circadian rhythm.

Morning light exposure acts as a powerful signal to our circadian clock, which resides in the brain and governs the timing of various bodily functions, including the sleep-wake cycle. Exposure to natural light in the morning helps reset this internal clock daily, ensuring it remains synchronized with the external 24-hour day-night cycle. This synchronization is vital for maintaining a consistent and healthy sleep pattern.

Furthermore, exposure to morning light has direct benefits on mood. The interaction with natural light, especially light rich in blue wavelengths, can uplift your mood and enhance overall well-being. This is particularly beneficial during menopause, a phase often marked by mood fluctuations and sleep disturbances.

Incorporating morning light exposure into your daily routine doesn't have to be complicated. It can be as simple as taking a short walk outside shortly after waking up, enjoying your morning coffee near a sunny window, or even doing some light stretching or yoga in a sunlit room. The key is to engage in activities that expose you to natural daylight, particularly within the first couple of hours after waking up, to help anchor your body's internal clock to the rhythm of the day.

By embracing morning light exposure as a natural tool to improve sleep quality, you're not just addressing a symptom of menopause – you're aligning your body's natural rhythm with the environment, setting a foundation for better overall health and well-being.

∼

Eat Well, Sleep Well

What you eat and drink can have a dramatic effect on the quality of your sleep. And a few simple tweaks could help you have a more restful night.

As mentioned earlier, watching out for stimulants such caffeine, which can stay in the body for up to seven hours after consumption. Try experimenting with timing your final hot drink of the day. Remember that dark chocolate is also high in caffeine so you may wish to avoid snacking on this late at night.

Many of us think that alcohol is a sedative but it actually increases dopamine in the brain which can be stimulating. It also disrupts blood sugar, as do other foods high in sugars like white rice, pasta, and sweet treats. This can lead to frequent waking and alter melatonin production, a hormone vital for your body's circadian rhythm.

Fluctuating estrogen levels can alter the amount of acid your stomach produces. 47% percent of menopausal women suffer from heartburn which is linked to poor sleep. Avoid spicy or fatty foods for dinner if this is an issue for you as they can lead to a build up of stomach acid which causes heartburn and discomfort.

Stick to regular meal times and try to have a diet that combines carbohydrates and protein which enables your body to make more of a sleep-inducing amino acid called tryptophan, that helps your brain make serotonin and melatonin for a better night's sleep.

Breathe Your Way to Blissful Sleep

You can use breath to help you switch off if you're anxious and find it hard to fall asleep and to get back to sleep if you wake up in the middle of the night. One of the most researched techniques to help you shift your nervous system from action to rest mode is the four-six-two breathing method. Where the numbers refer to the length of each step of breath: four counts inhale, six counts exhale, two counts pause.

A great breathing technique developed by sleep expert Dr Andrew Weil is called four-seven-eight breathing and is so simple. Place the tip of the tongue behind the front teeth, then exhale completely with whoosh sound, close your mouth, inhale through the nose for a count of four, hold your breath for seven and exhale for a count of eight with whoosh through your mouth. Repeat this cycle three times. You will notice that you get sleepy quickly.

∽

Creating the Perfect Bedroom

Sometimes, these issues really can just be fixed by making some basic tweaks to your sleeping environment. A conducive sleep environment is key to improving sleep quality:

- Optimal Room Temperature: Keeping the room cool can counteract night sweats and aid in falling asleep faster. The ideal temperature is generally between 60-67 degrees Fahrenheit (15.6-19.4 degrees Celsius).
- Utilizing Blackout Curtains: A dark environment cues the brain for sleep. Blackout curtains can significantly improve sleep quality, especially for light-sensitive individuals.
- Noise Management: Earplugs or a white noise machine can be effective, especially if you live in a noisy environment.
- Creating Comfort: Ensure your mattress and pillows are comfortable, and consider using breathable, moisture-wicking bedding to help with night sweats. Also consider cooling and moisture wicking nightwear. If you struggle with night sweats it can be

helpful to have a glass of water and a change of clothing close to hand.
- Leave Tech Out of the Bedroom: Combinations of blue light and constant information diminish the quality of sleep. Resist taking up your phone or laptop or turning on the TV if you are struggling to fall asleep to wake up in the night. This leave will make it hard to fall asleep and leave you feeling more tired the next day.

Creating A Routine for Better Sleep

- Consistent Sleep Schedule: Going to bed and waking up at the same time every day, even on weekends, helps to regulate your body's internal clock and improves the quality of your sleep.
- Relaxing Pre-Sleep Routine: Develop a calming routine before bed to signal to your body that it's time to wind down. This could include activities like reading, listening to soft music, light stretching, or a warm bath.
- Managing Blue Light Exposure: Exposure to blue light from screens can disrupt the body's production of melatonin, a hormone that regulates sleep. Limiting screen time in the evening and considering the use of blue light filtering glasses can help.
- Stay Calm in the Daytime: Keeping stress levels low in the day will help you sleep at night. Take breaks during your working day to relax and stretch. Even using scents and essential oils like lavender can calm, soothe and energize you throughout the day.

CONCLUSION

In menopause, managing sleep requires a holistic approach; recognizing the far-reaching implications of sleep on both physical and mental health is crucial. From unraveling the tangled web of hormonal shifts to shining a light on lifestyle habits and stressors, we've armed ourselves with the knowledge to reclaim our nights.

Chapter Takeaways:

- Decreased levels of estrogen and progesterone during menopause disrupt sleep patterns, leading to insomnia and night sweats.
- Additional factors impacting sleep include stress, anxiety, lifestyle habits, and health conditions like sleep apnea or restless leg syndrome.
- Make your bedroom a sanctuary for sleep by maintaining a cool temperature, using blackout curtains, and reducing noise.
- Practice good sleep hygiene by establishing regular sleep schedules, create relaxing pre-sleep routines, and limit exposure to blue light before bedtime.
- Incorporating deep breathing exercises, progressive muscle relaxation, gentle yoga, or guided meditation can help to prepare your mind and body for sleep.
- Increased anxiety during menopause can lead to a state of hyper-alertness at night, similar to a meerkat on guard. Stress management promotes good sleep.
- Embrace the role of morning light in setting your circadian rhythm. Engage in activities that expose you to natural daylight soon after waking.

Recommended listening for this chapter, from the Thriving Thru Menopause Podcast:

- Season 5 Episode 20: Sleep and Menopause
- Season 3 Episode 18: How to Sleep Better in Menopause

Scan This QR Code To Listen On Your Favorite Podcast App

SEXUAL HEALTH & INTIMACY

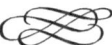

*S*ex is over in menopause is the biggest myth! But it doesn't have to be that way.

Menopause can bring with it changes in libido. But it is important to recognize that not every woman experiences a drop in libido, for some it can go crazy. This is both hormonal and later into perimenopause and early menopause there can also be a relief that we no longer can get pregnant, something that lives in the back of our minds.

But for many there is a drop in libido and various changes and lifestyle factors can affect your sex life around and after menopause. Factors that contribute to a fall in libido may include:

- Hormonal changes
- Physical changes
- Socio-psychological factors

Until recently this was an area that was taboo but with more fem-tech businesses providing products, healthcare and 'sexperts' speaking out on social media there is growing awareness that this an area that can be treated with understanding, and by adapting, and embracing a new approach to intimacy.

As well as the physical side it also requires an understanding of the ebbs and flows of libido and sexual response and an appreciation for the complexity of the changes your body and mind are undergoing.

UNDERSTANDING CHANGES IN LIBIDO AND SEXUAL RESPONSE DURING MENOPAUSE

You might notice that your libido, or sex drive, is changing. Some women may experience an increase in libido, while others experience a decrease. Not all women go through this libido decrease, though it is very common. In most cases, a lower libido during menopause is due to decreased hormone levels, your testosterone and estrogen levels both decrease, which may make it more difficult for you to get aroused.

In a recent survey of over 100K women 60% of women in menopause and early postmenopause report that sex is painful and that they are suffering with vaginal dryness. More than 40% of women report that penetrative sex is painful.

A decrease in estrogen can also lead to vaginal dryness. Lower levels of estrogen lead to a drop in blood supply in the vagina, which can then negatively affect vaginal lubrication. It can also lead to thinning of the vaginal wall, known as vaginal atrophy. As well as thinning of the labia, which leads to it becoming less sensitive to sexual stimulation.

Vaginal dryness and atrophy often lead to discomfort during sex. Painful sex is considered by many women to be one of the most severe symptoms of menopause. When combined with reduced blood flow may affect overall arousal. Sex may be less enjoyable, and it may be harder to have an orgasm.

But it isn't just changes in the vagina and vulva that might also affect your libido. Stress is one the biggest factors contributing to a drop in libido. Perimenopausal women are juggling a lot, more than we admit and can be highly stressed and used to putting more and more onto our to do list. And Mother Nature is wise, she prioritizes survival over reproduction and our hormones production then tilt towards cortisol and not our sex hormones. Hence the libido plummets.

Other menopausal symptoms such as hot flashes and night sweats can make you feel uncomfortable. While insomnia and fatigue that plague so many leaves us feeling too tired for sex. Other symptoms include mood symptoms, especially depression and anxiety, which can affect your sex drive. Changes in our weight or body shape can make us feel self-conscious, only 3% of midlife women report being totally comfortable with their bodies.

STRATEGIES FOR MAINTAINING SEXUAL HEALTH AND INTIMACY

Now that we have a better grasp on what changes to expect and why, let's talk about maintaining sexual health and intimacy during menopause. Because let's face it, nobody wants this vibrant part of life to fade away. It's all about finding the right balance and being open to adjustments.

When it comes to addressing discomfort in the vaginal area, starting with natural options, vaginal moisturizers containing hyaluronic acid are a top pick. Hyaluronic acid, a naturally occurring substance in our bodies, is known for its incredible ability to retain moisture. When used in vaginal moisturizers, it acts like a hydrating agent for your vaginal tissues, providing long-lasting moisture and relief from dryness. Regular use of these moisturizers can make a significant difference, not just in alleviating dryness but also in enhancing overall comfort during day-to-day activities and intimate moments. They're like a soothing balm, offering gentle, yet effective relief.

On the medical front, vaginal estrogen therapies are a powerful option. I can personally attest to how great a difference this has made to my vaginal tissues over the last few years. As you navigate through menopause, your body's estrogen levels drop, which is a primary cause of vaginal dryness and discomfort. Vaginal estrogen therapies work by locally administering estrogen directly to the vaginal area. This localized approach means that the therapy specifically targets the area in need, helping to restore the natural balance and health of the vaginal tissues. It's akin to replenish a depleted soil with essential nutrients, allowing the natural flora to thrive again. These therapies come in various forms, such as creams, tablets, or rings, and can significantly improve vaginal health by restoring moisture, elasticity, and comfort.

Lubricants, for instance, can reduce friction during intercourse, making the experience more enjoyable and less painful. You have options ranging from water-based and silicone-based lubricants to natural oil-based ones. Each type has its benefits, so you might want to experiment a bit to find what works best for you.

Besides lubricants, other aids like vaginal moisturizers, which are used regularly, can help maintain moisture levels in the vaginal area, providing longer-term relief from dryness. These aren't just for use during sexual activity; they're part of your daily vaginal health routine.

Of course there are also vibrators and other sexual devices. They aren't just for pleasure; they're therapeutic tools in their own right. They can stimulate blood flow to the vaginal area, which is essential for tissue health. Plus, they can be a fantastic way to explore your body and understand what feels good, which can change during menopause.

NAVIGATING VAGINAL HEALTH AND ITS IMPACT ON INTIMACY

An area of vaginal health that has been attracting more interest lately is the vaginal microbiome. Your vagina like your gut and skin, has a microbiome that might sound clinical, but it's essentially the community of microorganisms living in your vaginal area. The vagina, in its intricate balance, maintains a normal pH that is slightly acidic, typically ranging between 3.8 to 4.5. This acidity is crucial for its health, primarily maintained by lactobacilli, a type of beneficial bacteria. These microorganisms play a pivotal role in keeping harmful bacteria at bay, ensuring a healthy vaginal environment.

As estrogen levels fluctuate and eventually decline, so does the presence of lactobacilli, leading to changes in the vaginal pH. This shift can make the vagina less acidic and more susceptible to infections and discomfort. You may notice changes in moisture levels, leading to dryness, or an altered scent, which are signs of this shifting balance. But it's not just hormonal changes that impact this delicate ecosystem, many factors contribute to the health of your vaginal microbiome.

Sexual activity, for instance, can introduce new bacteria or alter the pH. It is advisable to use condoms if you have a new sexual partner for the first few months.

The vagina is self-cleaning so the products you use, ranging from soaps and lotions to douches and lubricants, can also have a significant impact. This means you should avoid douching – trying to clean inside the vagina – because it can harm this balance, or exacerbate an existing problem. The vulva, on the outside, can be cleaned "with water and a mild soap only".

Even your menstrual cycle, though it changes character during perimenopause and eventually ceases, can influence the vaginal pH. This isn't a mere inconvenience; it can deeply affect your comfort and pleasure during sex, impacting your desire and overall enjoyment.

Understanding your body's unique signals during this time is essential. Each woman's menopausal experience is different, so being aware of changes in scent, discharge, and appearance is vital. These aren't flaws but rather your body's way of adapting to its new hormonal environment. By tuning into these signals, you can approach these changes thoughtfully and effectively.

The vaginal microbiome may be regulated by either oral probiotics formulated to balance the vaginal microbiome and support the vagina's natural defense system. It is very important to check the quality of these oral supplements as many are at best placebos. More recently there has been innovation around pH regulated Gel Sticks that let you rebalance healthy vaginal acidity (3.8-5.0 pH) preventing dysbiosis and supporting conditions for healthy flora to thrive. Your diet is a great inexpensive way to support healthy microbiomes in the body - gut, skin and the vagina. Ensuring that your diet includes pro and prebiotic foods can be very effective.

Pelvic Organ Prolapse, a condition in which pelvic muscles can no longer adequately support organs in the pelvic area, is common in women, whose prevalence increases with age. Up to 50% of women will develop pelvic organ prolapse (POP) over their lifetime. Hormonal changes at menopause are a key factor and it can lead to painful sex.

Increasingly women are looking towards non-invasive treatment options. Physical therapy focuses on pelvic floor rehabilitation, muscle strengthening, and relaxation as well as kegel exercises. Lifestyle changes, such as weight loss, improved diet, fluid intake and exercise, and learning good bowel and bladder habits can all improve symptoms.

GREAT SEX IS POSSIBLE IN MENOPAUSE AND WELL INTO LATER LIFE

All this info might make you feel as if sex might be becoming more of a hassle than it's worth during menopause. So an important point to mention is that incorporating sexual activity is actually a vital part of maintaining vaginal health and enhancing intimacy during menopause!

It's kind of like keeping a machine well-oiled and running smoothly. Regular sexual activity, whether with a partner or through self-stimulation, acts like a beneficial workout for your vaginal area. It boosts blood flow to the tissues down there, which is crucial for keeping them healthy, elastic, and vibrant. Increased blood flow not only nourishes the vaginal tissues but also helps maintain their elasticity and lubrication, countering the dryness and thinning that often come with menopause.

Now, I get it – the idea of sexual activity might be daunting if you're experiencing discomfort or dryness. That's where lubricants and other sexual aids play a significant role. These are not just accessories; they are essential tools that can significantly enhance comfort and pleasure.

But great sex is about more than your physiology. Our sense of connection can often go astray in the busyness of midlife. If we have a partner we can find ourselves on parallel tracks busy with work and family commitments and sex becomes less of a shared experience.

If our partners are male they may be going through andropause, which can lead to a drop in testosterone levels, sometimes low moods and with that a loss of libido leading to a double whammy when it comes to sex and intimacy.

If you have been in a relationship for many years, maybe your sex life has become mundane and you no longer experiment or talk about what gives pleasure. This is a time to explore and communicate what we enjoy. It starts with getting to know our own bodies. One sex coach even suggests that women regularly set aside a whole day for self-pleasuring and explore their bodies- she described this as ultimate self-care. The more we know our pleasure points the more we can communicate to our partners. Try using phrases like 'I would enjoy if ….' or 'when you do …can we have more of that'. In the bedroom we can explore 'outcourse' in place of intercourse, massage, kissing, oral sex, as ways to bring sensuality rather than sexuality into the bedroom.

Beginning to create rituals provides an opportunity to bring more intimacy and sensuality into our relationships. Rituals are repeated ways of engaging with each other that carry a positive emotional component that distinguishes them from a routine. They can be small but the accumulative effect is potent. Try setting up some gentle rituals that are easy to do and cultivate the habit of laughter, playfulness and touch: Some examples include leaving some love notes or sending some flirty texts. Make being present to each other a priority. Consider a few minutes of connecting conversation rather than problem-solving any issues.

CONCLUSION

The sizzle of sexual attraction will ebb and flow but friendship, respect, fun and loving intention, can be the path to restoring or building intimacy and sensuality. Be creative and put your imagination to positive use and reclaim that loving, sensual feeling. Sex in menopause and beyond into our 70s and 80s can be deeply enjoyable. Pleasure is your right. A woman in her pleasure is a force of nature.

Chapter Takeaways:

- Recognize that decreased levels of estrogen and testosterone during menopause affect our libido levels and the health of our vagina.
- Additional factors impacting in particular stress, but also insomnia, fatigue, weight gain and anxiety all can significantly impact our desire to have sex.
- Personal lubricants and moisturizers are effective at relieving discomfort and pain during sexual intercourse for women with mild to moderate vaginal dryness. While locally applied estrogen creams and suppositories are very effective treatments for vaginal atrophy that are safe at low dose.
- The vagina is a self-cleaning organ. Avoid douching and clean the vulva, on the outside with water and a mild soap only. Probiotics either taken as supplements or introducing more fermented foods, such as sauerkraut, kimchi, kefir and kombucha, can help maintain a healthy vaginal microbiome.
- Incorporate kegel exercises or using devices that help to strengthen the pelvic floor are highly recommended. If you are experiencing issues then a visit to a pelvic floor physiotherapist should be your first point of call.
- Menopause is a time of change and it is vital to communicate what is going on for you with your partner and not feel pressured into having sex or having sex that is painful. As we age sexuality can give way to sensuality. It is time to explore what gives you pleasure.

Recommended listening for this chapter, from the Thriving Thru Menopause Podcast:

- Season 2 Episode 23 Have the Sex Life YOU want.
- Season 3 Episode 5 Making Sense of Menopause: Sexuality and Relationships.
- Season 3 Episode 26 Vaginal Health in Menopause
- Season 5 Episode 11 Pelvic Floor Problems in Menopause are Common, NOT normal and Can Be Solved

Scan This QR Code To Listen On Your Favorite Podcast App

POSITIVE AGING THROUGH MENOPAUSE

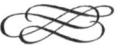

This book has been dedicated to providing you holistic ways to thrive through menopause, each chapter focusing on a different aspect. But amongst strategic approaches to diet, sleep, sexual health and more, there's one missing piece we haven't covered yet - how we actually view aging and menopause as a whole. It's time to shift our perspective towards one of the most transformative periods in a woman's life. The journey through menopause is deeply personal, yet universally resonant. It's a transition that involves not just physiological changes but also psychological, emotional, and societal shifts. Imagine a caterpillar's metamorphosis into a butterfly – intricate, detailed, with time spent in a messy mush before remerging transformed. Far from being merely an end to fertility, menopause offers a profound opportunity for introspection, self-discovery, and personal growth, but that's definitely not how it's portrayed in the modern world. This chapter is dedicated to embracing this transition, viewing it as an opportunity for self-discovery and a redefinition of roles in society.

THE MODERN MENOPAUSE DILEMMA

This period of life is a call to reconnect with ourselves, to evaluate and redefine what truly brings us fulfillment and joy, beyond societal expectations and external validations. Yet it often feels more so like a marker of aging, a point at which society suggests a woman's value, vitality, and visibility begin to wane. But why is this the case, when it doesn't need to be this way?

The roots of this perception are deep, tangled in historical misconceptions and a cultural obsession with youth. In a world that often values women for our fertility and physical appearance, menopause has been unfairly branded as a decline from a peak, rather than what it can truly be: an ascent to a new plateau of understanding, ability, and self-awareness.

Yet, this narrative is slowly but surely beginning to change. As more women speak out about their experiences, as more information becomes available, and as society begins to value diversity in all its forms, including age, the story of menopause is being rewritten. We're starting to see it not as an ending but as a powerful new beginning.

Globally, the number of post-menopausal women is growing. In 2021, women aged 50 and over accounted for 26% of all women and girls worldwide, up from 22% 10 years earlier.

From Belgium to Brazil to Bangladesh, women are pushing back against the stigma, dealing with symptoms, menopause often carries with it a bundle of negative connotations, a stigma that's been perpetuated through myths, misunderstandings, and a general lack of open, honest conversation about what it truly means to transition through this phase of life.

In traditional cultures, the onset of menopause used to signal not the end of a woman's vitality but the beginning of a new, esteemed chapter. It ushered in a phase where a woman steps into a role brimming with authority and respect. This role was not bestowed lightly; it was earned through years of life experience, wisdom, and the accumulated knowledge that comes with age. Eldership in these societies was not just a title; but a responsibility. Women in this stage of life were often turned to for advice, for conflict resolution, and for leading community ceremonies, reflecting their pivotal role in the cultural and spiritual life of the community.

This celebration of menopause contrasts sharply with the often negative framing in modern societies, where aging, particularly for women, is something to be combated, concealed, or lamented. Yet, in the traditional context, aging was embraced as a natural, honored progression of life. Here, menopause was not a quiet fading away but a vibrant step into greater visibility and influence within the community. It was a time when a woman's voice grew stronger, her words carried more weight, and her presence is a source of comfort and guidance for those around her.

This traditional view of menopause and aging presents a powerful counter-narrative to the modern perception. It's a reminder that the value and potential of women do not diminish with age. Instead, this transition can be a doorway to a period of life rich with opportunities for leadership, mentorship, and continued personal growth. It underscores the idea that menopause, far from being a decline, can be a moment of ascent - a time when the qualities a woman has honed over a lifetime come to the forefront, allowing her to assume a role of greater significance in her community.

Similarly, in the rich tapestry of traditional Indian culture, menopause was embraced as a significant and natural phase in a woman's life, mirroring the holistic and integrative approach to health and well-being that has been a cornerstone of this society for centuries. This perspective is deeply rooted in the wisdom of Ayurveda, an ancient healthcare system that sees menopause not as an ailment to be treated, but as a critical life stage that offers an opportunity for renewal and self-care.

Ayurveda teaches that life is a series of cycles and transitions, each with its own beauty and challenges. Menopause, in this context, is considered a vital transition, marking a shift from the childbearing years to a period of wisdom and introspection. It's a time when a woman's energies are believed to realign, presenting an opportunity to focus inward and nurture the soul as well as the body.

The Ayurvedic approach to menopause is highly personalized, recognizing that each woman experiences this transition uniquely. By understanding one's 'dosha' or body type - Vata, Pitta, or Kapha - Ayurvedic practitioners tailor interventions that promote balance and health during menopause. Dietary adjustments are central to this, with a focus on foods that nourish and support the body's changing needs. Herbal supplements, too, play a crucial role, offering natural remedies to ease symptoms and support overall well-being.

Lifestyle changes are also advocated, encouraging practices like yoga and meditation to harmonize the body and spirit. These practices are not just about physical health but are seen as essential for emotional and spiritual well-being, helping to navigate the menopausal transition with grace and ease.

According to traditional Chinese culture a woman's menstrual life is like halves of the moon. When she reaches midlife the body and mind are naturally ready to explore another half-phase of the moon. Perimenopause and menopause mark the time that the transition begins - wake up call to focus on change in a positive and healthy way.

The hormone imbalances caused by menopause should neither be the culprit that women blame for all their health problems nor the root of their overall health. Post menopause the mind is calmer and energy and creativity rise to greet what is termed the Second Spring.

In this way, Ayurvedic and Chinese contexts offer profoundly positive and empowering views of menopause. It's seen as a time of growth, a stage of life where women are encouraged to explore and embrace their inner strength, wisdom, and vitality.

THE IMPACT OF SOCIETAL STEREOTYPES

In the midst of menopause, the physical and emotional transformations you undergo can test your self-esteem. It's a time when society's long-held stereotypes - that youth alone is beautiful and that vitality fades with age - can unfairly color your self-perception. These societal messages are pervasive, creeping into our thoughts and silently shaping how we view ourselves during this significant life transition. The challenge, then, is to consciously and actively dismantle these harmful notions, replacing them with a more compassionate and self-affirming outlook.

Society often paints aging, especially for women, in a negative light. Media and cultural messages bombard us with the idea that menopause is a period of loss - loss of fertility, loss of youth, and by erroneous extension, loss of relevance and attractiveness. This narrative can deeply affect how we perceive ourselves as women during menopause, leading to feelings of invisibility or a diminished sense of value. Menopause emerges not as a period of decline but as a vibrant phase of transformation and renewal. It offers a profound opportunity for introspection and reconnection, inviting us to delve deep into the essence of who we are and who we wish to become. This stage of life beckons us to look beyond societal expectations and norms about aging, urging us to find value and fulfillment within ourselves rather than seeking external validation. It calls for an act of rebellion against these ingrained societal norms. It requires cultivating self-compassion and recognizing that the changes you're experiencing don't detract from your worth but add to the depth of your character. Aging is as natural as the seasons;

it's a process that brings its own kind of beauty, marked by wisdom, resilience, and a fuller sense of self.

Rejecting negative stereotypes involves rewriting the narrative around menopause and aging. It's about seeing menopause not as a period of decline but as a potent opportunity for personal growth and self-renewal. This period offers a chance to rediscover who you are, independent of societal roles or expectations. It invites you to evaluate what truly matters to you, to honor the wealth of experience you bring, and to redefine what fulfillment looks like at this stage in your life.

Rewriting the narrative about menopause and aging isn't just an abstract idea; it's a practical, day-to-day process that involves actively changing how we talk to and about ourselves. This means challenging and replacing the internalized messages that society has ingrained in us with more positive, empowering beliefs. Here's how you can start:

First, acknowledge how societal stereotypes about menopause and aging make you feel. It's okay to feel vulnerable, frustrated, or even angry. Recognizing these feelings is the first step toward changing the narrative, through cultivating a deep sense of self-awareness. Ask yourself what menopause means to you beyond the physical changes. What aspects of this transition are you grateful for? What strengths have you discovered in yourself? Reflecting on these questions can help shift your focus from loss to gain.

What does fulfillment look like for you at this stage of your life? It might be different from what it was twenty years ago, and that's perfectly okay. Perhaps it's pursuing a long-held passion, dedicating more time to relationships, or finding new ways to express your creativity. Define it on your own terms. Set intentions for how you want to experience this phase of your life. Intention setting is a powerful practice that can guide your actions and thoughts toward the positive narrative you're creating. These intentions can be as simple as practicing gratitude daily, exploring a new hobby, or nurturing your relationships. Something practical I'd recommend to try is every morning, write down 10 things you are grateful for. It doesn't matter what they are, just whatever comes to mind first. This may range from something as current as the weather to even gratitude towards the people that built your house (that you may have never met). This also helps as a way of actually reframing certain changes so you can embrace them. At the end of writing, say out loud 'thank you' 3 times. When we hear/say something 3 times or more, it helps absorb the information more and in this case, reaffirms the overall mood here much deeper in your subconscious. Do this for the next 28 days and see how you feel before and after!

Be kind to yourself. Practice self-compassion by speaking to yourself as you would to a dear friend going through the same transition. Remind yourself of your worth, your strengths, and the beauty of evolving into a more authentic version of yourself. This is especially important when actively challenging the societal messages that equate youth with value. When you encounter ageist stereotypes, whether in media, conversation, or even in your thoughts, question them. Remind yourself of the accomplishments, wisdom, and depth you've gained over the years that no younger version of yourself possessed.

Finally, celebrate your evolution. Menopause is a significant milestone that marks the passage into a new, potentially richer phase of life. Celebrate your growth, the wisdom you've accumulated, and the person you're becoming. Recognize that with this transition comes a powerful new role in your own life and in the lives of those around you.

By actively engaging in these practices, you can start to rewrite the narrative around menopause and aging. Letting go of societal stereotypes and negative self-talk opens the door to a more empowering view of menopause. It's an opportunity to embrace the changes, to grow, and to step into a new version of yourself with confidence. By doing so, you affirm that your value and beauty are not tied to youth but to the richness of your life's journey. Menopause, then, becomes not a time of waning but a time of blossoming into a more authentic and self-assured you.

In embracing this perspective, you not only enrich your own experience of menopause but also contribute to a broader cultural shift that recognizes the strength, beauty, and wisdom that come with aging. It's a step towards a society where menopause is celebrated as a significant life milestone, marked by personal growth, renewed purpose, and continued vitality. Again, the Western world is catching up with other cultures here!

SELF DISCOVERY THROUGH MENOPAUSE

The transition through menopause can be likened to a journey of self-discovery. It's a time when the noise of the world dims, allowing us to listen more closely to our inner voice. This phase encourages us to reflect on our experiences, the roles we've played, and the dreams we may have set aside. It's an invitation to explore new interests, revive forgotten passions, and perhaps, redefine our life's direction. The transformational aspect of menopause is not just about the physical changes our bodies undergo but about the emotional and spiritual growth that can flourish during this time.

Redefining personal significance and fulfillment during menopause means moving away from societal benchmarks of success and beauty and fostering a sense of worth that is deeply rooted in our own values and desires. It's about recognizing the richness of our experiences and the wisdom we've accumulated. This stage of life offers a unique vantage point from which to view our lives, providing clarity on what truly matters to us.

As we navigate this transition, it becomes crucial to cultivate a practice of self-care and self-love. This might mean setting boundaries, prioritizing our health, and making space for activities that bring us joy and rejuvenation. It's also a time to strengthen our relationships with those who support and uplift us, fostering connections that nourish our souls. While a noble ideal, it can feel like navigating uncharted waters. The societal benchmarks of success and beauty, deeply ingrained, do not vanish overnight. Here's how you can embark on this journey of redefinition and embrace this stage of life with confidence and grace.

- Reflect and Reassess: Take time to reflect on your life's journey so far. Journaling can be a powerful tool in this process, helping you to uncover your true values and desires. Ask yourself what truly brings you joy, fulfillment, and a sense of purpose. This might be different from what you've been conditioned to value.

- Cultivate Self-Care and Self-Love: Begin by establishing a routine that prioritizes your well-being. Being this far into the book, this should already be something top of mind for you and hopefully you have clarity on what this might look like; incorporating a balanced diet, regular physical activity, and practices like meditation or yoga that foster a connection between mind, body, and spirit. Remember, self-care is not selfish; it's necessary. By taking care of yourself, you're better equipped to explore new avenues of fulfillment and joy. Finding joy in small changes and embracing the fluid nature of life can also revitalize your outlook and self love. Celebrate the small victories, whether it's mastering a new recipe, finishing a book, or simply taking time for yourself each day. Acknowledge the progress in these seemingly insignificant actions; they're stepping stones towards larger goals and a testament to your resilience and adaptability.
- Set Boundaries: Learning to say no is a form of self-respect. Set boundaries that protect your energy and time, making space for activities and people that align with your values and bring you happiness. This might mean declining commitments that no longer serve you or stepping away from relationships that drain your spirit.
- Explore New Passions: Menopause is the perfect time to rediscover old interests or to explore new ones. Whether it's taking up painting, joining a dance

class, or volunteering for a cause close to your heart, engaging in activities that resonate with you can be incredibly fulfilling. It's about allowing yourself to explore without the pressure of excelling or meeting external expectations.

- Strengthen Your Support Network: Surround yourself with people who uplift and support you. This could mean deepening existing relationships or seeking out new communities that share your interests or are going through similar life stages. Remember, vulnerability in sharing your journey can lead to stronger, more meaningful connections.
- Embrace Change: Viewing menopause as an opportunity rather than a loss is pivotal. Embrace the changes happening within and around you, viewing each as a step toward a more authentic self. Change is inevitable, but how we respond to it can transform our lives in beautiful ways.
- Practice Gratitude: Cultivate a habit of gratitude. Focusing on the positives in your life, even the small victories or simple pleasures, can shift your perspective and help you find joy in the everyday. Gratitude can be a grounding force, reminding you of the abundance present in your life, even amidst transition. The exercise in this chapter is a great place to start!

By integrating these practices into your daily life, you'll find that redefining personal significance and fulfillment during menopause is not only possible but can be a deeply rewarding experience. Start with small, achievable goals that align with your interests and capabilities. This could be as simple as dedicating ten minutes a day to meditation or setting a weekly goal to connect with a friend. These actions build a foundation for larger achievements, fostering a sense of progress and fulfillment.

CONCLUSION

Like the metamorphosis of a caterpillar into a butterfly, we've seen menopause as a chance for introspection, self-discovery, and a redefinition of our roles within society. This transition, while deeply personal, echoes universally, resonating with the shared experiences of women across the globe. Drawing inspiration from traditional cultures, we've reimagined menopause as a time of esteemed change, where women step into roles of authority and wisdom, celebrated for their experience and knowledge.

Ultimately, maintaining vitality and energy through menopause isn't about grand gestures or overhauling your life overnight. It's about recognizing the power of incremental changes and the value of nurturing your well-being on every level.

This stage of life is not about diminishing but about blossoming into a fuller, more realized version of yourself. Embracing menopause and aging as positive, empowering stages of life allows us to shift our focus from societal expectations to finding internal satisfaction and purpose.

Chapter Takeaways:

- Embrace the transition through menopause as a vibrant step into greater visibility, influence, and a role brimming with authority and respect, contrary to the modern portrayal of this life stage as a decline in value and vitality.
- There's a growing global conversation around menopause, where women from diverse cultures push back against stigma and embrace this phase as a powerful blossoming into a more authentic and self-assured individual, contributing to a broader cultural shift that celebrates the strength, beauty, and wisdom that come with aging.
- Draw inspiration from traditional views of menopause, like in Ayurvedic and Chinese cultures, where it's seen as a natural, honored progression of life, emphasizing growth, wisdom, and vitality.
- Actively reject and rewrite the negative narratives surrounding menopause and aging by fostering a sense of worth rooted in personal values and experiences, challenging the societal equating of youth with value.
- Pursue self-discovery by redefining personal significance and fulfillment during menopause, focusing on what truly brings joy and satisfaction beyond societal benchmarks of success and beauty.
- Integrate nutrition, physical activity, and mindful practices into daily life as part of a holistic approach to thriving through menopause, focusing on incremental changes and the power of nurturing well-being on every level.

Recommended listening for this chapter, from the Thriving Thru Menopause Podcast:

- Season 3 Episode 14 The Upgrade: How the Female Brain Get Stronger and Better in Midlife and Beyond
- Season 3 Episode 3: Rebranding Midlife and Menopause
- Season 4 Episode 1 Revolutionsing Midlife

Scan This QR Code To Listen On Your Favorite Podcast App

CONCLUSION

Menopause, as we've discovered, isn't a solitary journey but a shared experience, a universal passage that connects us to the wisdom of generations before and the promise of those to come. It's a reminder that our bodies are not betraying us but simply moving into a new rhythm, a new way of being that calls for celebration, not concealment.

As you reflect on the chapters, think of them not just as sections of a book but as facets of a journey - a journey that's uniquely yours yet universally understood. Each chapter, from understanding the physical changes to mastering the art of positive aging, is a step towards embracing menopause with confidence and joy.

We've explored a ton of options for managing menopause symptoms, from nutritional strategies to mind-body practices and optimising your sleep. That's a lot, isn't it? You

CONCLUSION

might be wondering, "How do I choose what's right for me?" Well, let's put it this way: think of your menopause management as crafting your unique wellness recipe. You don't need every ingredient on the shelf - just the ones that resonate with your needs.

So, how do you decide? First, consider what symptoms are most pressing for you. If hot flashes are your main concern, you might lean towards understanding your food and stress triggers and seeing how you could change those. Struggling with mood swings? Look at ways you reduce your stress and create more emotional balance. This is where mind-body practices such as yoga or mindfulness meditation or more formal support in the CBT could be your go-to.

It's also important to consider your lifestyle. If you're always on the go, carrying a small bottle of peppermint oil for a quick pick-me-up might be a practical way to make a quick improvement. Or, if you find joy in quiet evenings at home, setting aside time for meditation or a yoga routine could be a perfect fit. Another key factor is your personal philosophy and comfort level. Are you drawn more to traditional, natural remedies? Medicinal herbs and essential oils might speak to your soul. Or, do you prefer structured practices that also offer physical benefits? Then tai chi or yoga might be more up your alley.

The beauty of this journey is that it's deeply personal. You don't have to do everything. Start by picking one or two methods that resonate with you the most. Give them a try, observe how your body and mind respond, and then adjust as needed. It's okay to experiment and switch things up. What works for one woman in menopause might not work for another - and that's perfectly fine. This book isn't about overwhelming you with options; it's about empowering you with choices. It's about finding what aligns with your unique menopausal journey. So, take a deep breath, listen to your body, and let your intuition guide you. This is your journey, and you have the power to choose the path that feels right for you.

Let's imagine you're someone who faces frequent hot flashes and stress, and you have a moderately busy lifestyle. Your daily routine might look something like this:

Morning

Start your day with some yoga stretches. These will encourage your brain to wake up even if you have had a restless night and raise your energy levels.

Making time to step outside in the morning may feel like a luxury, but prioritizing outdoor time first thing can have a positive impact on your entire day. It will regulate circadian rhythms so you sleep better, increase serotonin which is good for managing those menopause moods and morning sunlight has been shown to improve focus, concentration and productivity which is a bonus if brain fog is one of your symptoms.

Incorporate protein in your breakfast, try swapping a cereal or toast for Greek yogurt and some berries and don't forget to add a tablespoon of ground flax seeds which is rich in phytoestrogens, and can contribute to maintaining a healthy weight.

Midday

Keep a small bottle of peppermint essential oil at your desk or in your bag. If you feel a wave of fatigue or a hot flash coming on, a quick whiff can be refreshing and energizing.

Make time for a short walk at lunch time or park in the far spot in the car park and get those extra steps in. See if you can work extra movement into your day. Working standing up can burn more calories and strengthen your leg and core muscles. And anything you can do while walking around, do it. I always walk around on business calls unless I have to be closely looking at a document.

Take regular short breaks throughout the day to cope with brain fog in the workplace to rest your mind and recharge. You

can support this further by opting for lunch that is rich in antioxidants that are vital for brain health. The richest sources of antioxidants are in brightly coloured vegetables and fruits.

Evening

With dinner, try a side of pickles or kimchi to actively include additional probiotics in your diet, to promote a healthy gut and therefore better manage symptoms such as hot flashes.

Create an evening ritual that helps you transition from the day to night with minimum stress. Try some gentle breathwork and aim for digital detox at least 30 minutes before bed. If your head is swirling with thoughts, try writing down any worries. Also jot down three positive things that happened to your day and three things you are grateful for. Notice how this changes the quality of your mood and helps you focus on constructive thoughts rather than letting anxiety take hold.

Hopefully these examples show you how different methods can complement each other and fit into various parts of your day. You might find that certain practices resonate more with you than others, and that's okay. The key is to listen to your body and adjust accordingly. This journey through menopause is unique for each of us, and the beauty lies in discovering what works best for you. Let's recap how you can practically go from reading this book and all the ideas discussed, to actually having a day-to-day where you feel happier, look forward to these new holistic parts of your routine, and of course reap the amazing mental and physical benefits these natural solutions have to offer:

- Crafting a Personal Holistic Routine: Menopause, as we know, isn't a one-size-fits-all experience. It's a personal journey, and that's why incorporating holistic ways into our daily lives requires a bit of trial and error to find what resonates with us individually. The key is to build a routine that feels less like a chore and more like a cherished part of your day and that can be sustained even when life feels challenging.
- Starting Small and Being Consistent: Begin by introducing small, manageable practices into your routine. It could be as simple as starting your day with a protein rich breakfast. Or getting some extra daily movement into your day beyond your

scheduled gym session. The trick is to be consistent. Consistency is what builds habits, and over time, these small practices can lead to significant changes in how you manage menopausal symptoms.
- Listening to Your Body: Pay attention to how your body and mind feels when you make small changes. Maybe a short bedtime ritual, or perhaps a few minutes of meditation at your desk bring a sense of calmness. This feedback is crucial in tailoring a routine that works specifically for you.
- Combining Therapies for Synergy: Think about combining different approaches for a synergistic effect. For example, pairing aromatherapy with meditation can enhance the relaxation experience. Or, integrating regularly standing on one leg while you brush teeth alongside your strength training can help in maintaining healthy bones.
- Adjusting as You Go: As you progress through perimenopause into menopause and the next chapter of life your needs may change, and so should your holistic routine. Don't hesitate to adjust or swap out things as your body evolves. The goal is to support yourself through this transition in the most comfortable and effective way possible.
- Creating a Supportive Environment: Finally, consider your environment. Is it conducive to the practices you're adopting? Sometimes, creating a small, dedicated space for meditation or yoga can make a big difference. Surround yourself with elements that promote relaxation and well-being, like soothing colors, comfortable cushions, or even just a corner with your favorite plants.

Remember, thriving through menopause doesn't require perfection. It's about making choices that resonate with you, that bring you comfort, energy, and happiness. It's about tuning into your body, honoring its wisdom, and navigating the changes with grace and curiosity.

And as we bring this conversation to a close, let's carry with us the understanding that menopause is not just a phase to get through but a significant life stage to live fully. It's an opportunity to lean into the changes, to explore what truly matters, and to emerge with a renewed sense of purpose and passion.

BIBLIOGRAPHY

Alcohol questions and answers (2022) *Centers for Disease Control and Prevention.* Available at: https://www.cdc.gov/alcohol/faqs.htm#:

Covassin, Naima; Singh, Prachi; McCrady-Spitzer, Shelly; u. a. (2022): „Effects of experimental sleep restriction on Energy Intake, energy expenditure, and visceral obesity". *Journal of the American College of Cardiology.* Elsevier Abgerufen am 17.02.2024 von https://www.sciencedirect.com/science/article/pii/S0735109722003102?via=ihub.

Hairston, K.G. *et al.* (2012a) 'Lifestyle factors and 5-year abdominal fat accumulation in a minority cohort: The iras family study', *Obesity*, 20(2), pp. 421–427. doi:10.1038/oby.2011.171.

Khan, N.A. *et al.* (2021b) *Avocado consumption, abdominal adiposity, and oral glucose tolerance among persons with overweight and obesity*, The Journal of Nutrition. Available at: https://www.sciencedirect.com/science/article/pii/S0022316622003200?via%3Dihub

Martin, H. (no date) *4 easy low-carb diet meal plans from Dietitians*, TODAY.com. Available at: https://www.today.com/health/diet-fitness/low-carb-diet-meal-plan-foods-rcna34580

Morris, M.C. (2023) *Diet Review: Mind diet, The Nutrition Source.* Available at: https://www.hsph.harvard.edu/nutritionsource/healthy-weight/diet-reviews/mind-diet/

R., J.A. *et al.* (2011) *Increased consumption of dairy foods and protein during diet- and exercise-induced weight loss promotes fat mass loss and lean mass gain in overweight and obese premenopausal women*, The Journal of Nutrition. Available at: https://www.sciencedirect.com/science/article/pii/S0022316622030516?via=ihub

Salleh, Siti Nurshabani *et al.* (2019) 'Unravelling the effects of soluble dietary fibre supplementation on energy intake and perceived satiety in healthy adults: Evidence from systematic review and meta-analysis of randomised-controlled trials', *Foods*, 8(1), p. 15. doi:10.3390/foods8010015.

Kristjansson, C. (2018-2024) *Thriving Thru Menopause*. [Podcast]. Available at: Apple Podcasts.

www.ingramcontent.com/pod-product-compliance
Lightning Source LLC
LaVergne TN
LVHW041609070526
838199LV00052B/3064